Nourish to Flourish: Empowering Your Cancer Journey

Evelyn Sterling

Chapter 1: *Understanding* Cancer

Cancer is a complex disease that affects millions of people around the world. It is a leading cause of death, and the number of cancer cases is expected to continue to rise in the coming years. Despite the prevalence of cancer, many people do not fully understand what cancer is, how it develops, and how it can be prevented.

At its core, cancer is a group of diseases characterized by the uncontrolled growth and spread of abnormal cells. These cells can invade surrounding tissues and organs, leading to serious health problems and even death. There are many different types of cancer, each with its own unique characteristics, risk factors, and treatment options.

In this chapter, we will explore the basics of cancer, including its causes, symptoms, diagnosis, and treatment. We will also discuss some of the risk factors for cancer, such as lifestyle factors, genetics, and environmental exposures. By gaining a better understanding of cancer, we can take steps to reduce our risk of developing the disease and detect it early when treatment is most effective.

While cancer can be a devastating diagnosis, it is important to remember that there is hope. Advances in cancer research and treatment have led to improved survival rates and quality of life for many people with cancer. With knowledge and awareness, we can work together to prevent cancer and improve the lives of those affected by this disease.

What is cancer?

Cancer is a complex disease that can arise in any part of the body. At its core, cancer is a group of diseases characterized by the uncontrolled growth and spread of abnormal cells. Unlike normal cells in the body, cancer cells do not follow the usual growth and division patterns. Instead, they continue to divide and grow uncontrollably, often forming a mass of tissue known as a tumor. Tumors can be either benign or malignant. Benign tumors are not cancerous and do not spread to other parts of the body. They may still require treatment if they grow large enough to cause problems, but they are not life-threatening. Malignant tumors, on the other hand, are cancerous and can spread to other parts of the body through a process called metastasis. Metastasis occurs when cancer cells break away from the original tumor and travel through the bloodstream or lymphatic system to form new tumors in other parts of the body.

There are many different types of cancer, each with its own unique characteristics and risk factors. Some of the most common types of cancer include breast cancer, lung cancer, prostate cancer, and colorectal cancer. Other less common types of cancer include leukemia, lymphoma, and melanoma. The causes of cancer are complex and can involve a combination of genetic, environmental, and lifestyle factors. Some genetic mutations can increase the risk of developing certain types of cancer, while environmental factors such as exposure to toxins or radiation can also increase the risk. Lifestyle factors such as tobacco use, poor diet, and lack of exercise can also contribute to the development of cancer.

The symptoms of cancer can vary depending on the type of cancer and the stage of the disease. Some common symptoms of cancer include fatigue, unexplained weight loss, pain, and changes in the skin or the appearance of a lump or swelling. It is important to note that not all symptoms are indicative of cancer, and many other conditions can cause similar symptoms. That's why it's important to seek medical attention if you experience any unusual or persistent symptoms.

In summary, cancer is a complex disease characterized by the uncontrolled growth and spread of abnormal cells. It can arise in any part of the body and can be either benign or malignant. The causes of cancer are complex and can involve a combination of genetic, environmental, and lifestyle factors. Early detection and treatment are crucial for improving the prognosis of cancer, so it's important to stay informed and aware of the signs and symptoms of the disease.

Types of cancer

Bladder cancer:

Bladder cancer is a type of cancer that begins in the cells that line the inside of the bladder. It typically affects older adults, and it is more common in men than in women. There are several different types of bladder cancer, including transitional cell carcinoma, squamous cell carcinoma, and adenocarcinoma. Transitional cell carcinoma is the most common type of bladder cancer.

Risk factors for bladder cancer include:

- Smoking: Smoking is the most significant risk factor for bladder cancer. Smokers are more than twice as likely as non-smokers to develop bladder cancer.

- Exposure to certain chemicals: Exposure to certain chemicals, such as aromatic amines, can increase the risk of bladder cancer. These chemicals are found in many industrial products, including dyes, paints, and rubber products.

- Chronic bladder inflammation: Chronic bladder inflammation, caused by conditions such as urinary tract infections or bladder stones, can increase the risk of bladder cancer.

- Age and gender: Bladder cancer is more common in older adults and in men.
- Genetics: Some inherited genetic mutations can increase the risk of bladder cancer.

Symptoms of bladder cancer may include blood in the urine, pain during urination, and frequent urination. Treatment for bladder cancer depends on the stage and type of cancer, but it may include surgery, chemotherapy, or radiation therapy.

It's important to note that early detection and treatment of bladder cancer can improve the prognosis of the disease. If you experience any symptoms of bladder cancer, or if you have any concerns about your risk for bladder cancer, talk to your healthcare provider.

Brain and spinal cord tumors

Brain and spinal cord tumors are abnormal growths of cells in the brain or spinal cord. They can be benign (non-cancerous) or malignant (cancerous). Brain tumors can be primary (originating in the brain) or secondary (spreading from cancer in other parts of the body).

Risk factors for brain and spinal cord tumors include:

- Genetics: Certain inherited genetic conditions, such as neurofibromatosis, can increase the risk of developing brain and spinal cord tumors.

- Exposure to radiation: Exposure to high doses of ionizing radiation, such as radiation therapy for cancer treatment, can increase the risk of brain and spinal cord tumors.

- Age: Brain and spinal cord tumors are more common in older adults, although they can occur at any age.

- Gender: Certain types of brain tumors, such as meningiomas, are more common in women.

Symptoms of brain and spinal cord tumors can vary depending on the location and size of the tumor, but may include headaches, seizures, vision or hearing problems, difficulty with balance or coordination, and weakness or numbness in the limbs.

Treatment for brain and spinal cord tumors may include surgery, radiation therapy, chemotherapy, or a combination of these treatments. The type of treatment depends on the type and location of the tumor, as well as the patient's overall health.

It's important to note that early detection and treatment of brain and spinal cord tumors can improve the prognosis of the disease. If you experience any symptoms of a brain or spinal cord tumor, or if you have any concerns about your risk for these types of tumors, talk to your healthcare provider.

Breast cancer

Breast cancer is a type of cancer that begins in the breast tissue. It can occur in both men and women, but it is much more common in women. There are several different types of breast cancer, including ductal carcinoma in situ, invasive ductal carcinoma, and invasive lobular carcinoma.

Risk factors for breast cancer include:

- Age and gender: Breast cancer is more common in older women, and women are at a higher risk of developing breast cancer than men.

- Genetics: Certain inherited genetic mutations, such as BRCA1 and BRCA2, can increase the risk of developing breast cancer.

- Personal history of breast cancer: Women who have had breast cancer in one breast are at an increased risk of developing breast cancer in the other breast.
- Family history of breast cancer: Women who have a mother, sister, or daughter with breast cancer are at an increased risk of developing the disease.

- Hormonal factors: Factors that increase the amount of estrogen in the body, such as early onset of menstruation, late menopause, and never having been pregnant, can increase the risk of breast cancer.

Symptoms of breast cancer may include a lump or thickening in the breast tissue, changes in the shape or size of the breast, nipple discharge or inversion, and skin changes such as dimpling or redness.

Treatment for breast cancer depends on the type and stage of the cancer, but may include surgery, radiation therapy, chemotherapy, hormone therapy, or targeted therapy. Breast cancer screening, such as mammograms and clinical breast exams, can help with early detection of breast cancer.

It's important to note that early detection and treatment of breast cancer can improve the prognosis of the disease. If you experience any symptoms of breast cancer, or if you have any concerns about your risk for breast cancer, talk to your healthcare provider.

Cervical cancer

Cervical cancer is a type of cancer that begins in the cells lining the cervix, which is the lower part of the uterus that connects to the vagina. Cervical cancer is almost always caused by human papillomavirus (HPV) infection.

Risk factors for cervical cancer include:

- HPV infection: The most important risk factor for cervical cancer is HPV infection. HPV is a sexually transmitted infection that is very common, but most women who become infected with HPV do not develop cervical cancer.

- Smoking: Women who smoke are at an increased risk of developing cervical cancer.

- Weakened immune system: Women with weakened immune systems, such as those with HIV/AIDS or who have had an organ transplant, are at an increased risk of developing cervical cancer.

- Family history: Women who have a mother or sister who has had cervical cancer are at an increased risk of developing the disease.

- Symptoms of cervical cancer may include abnormal vaginal bleeding, such as bleeding between periods, after sex, or after menopause, as well as vaginal discharge, pelvic pain, and pain during sex.

Cervical cancer screening, such as the Pap test and HPV testing, can help with early detection of cervical cancer. The HPV vaccine can also help prevent HPV infection and reduce the risk of cervical cancer.

Treatment for cervical cancer depends on the type and stage of the cancer, but may include surgery, radiation therapy, chemotherapy, or a combination of these treatments.

Colorectal cancer

Colorectal cancer, also known as bowel cancer or colon cancer, is a type of cancer that begins in the colon or rectum. It typically develops slowly over several years, beginning as a small growth called a polyp.

Risk factors for colorectal cancer include:

- Age: Colorectal cancer is more common in older adults, with most cases occurring after the age of 50.

- Family history: Individuals with a family history of colorectal cancer or polyps are at an increased risk of developing the disease.

- Inherited syndromes: Certain genetic conditions, such as Lynch syndrome and familial adenomatous polyposis, can increase the risk of developing colorectal cancer.

- Lifestyle factors: A diet high in red meat and processed meats, a lack of physical activity, obesity, and smoking can increase the risk of developing colorectal cancer.

Symptoms of colorectal cancer may include changes in bowel habits, such as diarrhea, constipation, or narrowing of the stool, blood in the stool, abdominal pain, bloating, and fatigue.

Screening for colorectal cancer, such as colonoscopies, can help with early detection of the disease. Treatment for colorectal cancer depends on the stage and location of the cancer, but may include surgery, radiation therapy, chemotherapy, or a combination of these treatments.

Endometrial cancer

Endometrial cancer, also known as uterine cancer, is a type of cancer that begins in the lining of the uterus (endometrium). It is the most common type of cancer of the female reproductive system.

Risk factors for endometrial cancer include:

- Age: Endometrial cancer is more common in postmenopausal women, with most cases occurring after the age of 50.

- Obesity: Obesity is a significant risk factor for endometrial cancer, as it can lead to increased levels of estrogen in the body.

- Hormonal imbalances: Conditions that cause hormonal imbalances, such as polycystic ovary syndrome (PCOS) or estrogen replacement therapy without progesterone, can increase the risk of endometrial cancer.

- Family history: Women with a family history of endometrial cancer or certain inherited genetic conditions, such as Lynch syndrome, are at an increased risk of developing the disease.

Symptoms of endometrial cancer may include abnormal vaginal bleeding, such as bleeding between periods, after sex, or after menopause, as well as pelvic pain or pressure.

Endometrial cancer is typically diagnosed through a biopsy of the endometrial tissue. Treatment for endometrial cancer depends on the stage and location of the cancer, but may include surgery, radiation therapy, chemotherapy, or a combination of these treatments.

Esophageal cancer

Esophageal cancer is a type of cancer that occurs in the esophagus, which is the tube that connects the throat to the stomach. There are two main types of esophageal cancer: squamous cell carcinoma and adenocarcinoma.

Risk factors for esophageal cancer include:

- Tobacco use: Smoking or using other tobacco products can increase the risk of esophageal cancer.

- Alcohol consumption: Heavy alcohol consumption over a prolonged period can increase the risk of esophageal cancer.

- Gastroesophageal reflux disease (GERD): Chronic acid reflux, which can cause inflammation of the esophagus, can increase the risk of esophageal cancer.

- Barrett's esophagus: A condition in which the lining of the esophagus is damaged and replaced with abnormal cells, which can increase the risk of esophageal cancer.

- Obesity: Obesity can increase the risk of esophageal cancer, possibly due to increased levels of inflammation and acid reflux.

Symptoms of esophageal cancer may include difficulty swallowing, chest pain, weight loss, and regurgitation of food or fluids.

Esophageal cancer is typically diagnosed through a combination of imaging tests and biopsies. Treatment for esophageal cancer depends on the stage and location of the cancer, but may include surgery, radiation therapy, chemotherapy, or a combination of these treatments.

Gastric (stomach) cancer

Gastric (stomach) cancer is a type of cancer that occurs in the lining of the stomach. There are several types of gastric cancer, including adenocarcinoma, lymphoma, and gastrointestinal stromal tumor (GIST).

Risk factors for gastric cancer include:

- Helicobacter pylori infection: A bacterial infection of the stomach lining, which can lead to chronic inflammation, is a major risk factor for gastric cancer.

- Family history: People with a family history of gastric cancer are at an increased risk of developing the disease.

- Diet: A diet high in smoked or salted foods, as well as a lack of fruits and vegetables, can increase the risk of gastric cancer.

- Tobacco and alcohol use: Smoking or using other tobacco products, as well as heavy alcohol consumption, can increase the risk of gastric cancer.

Symptoms of gastric cancer may include abdominal pain, bloating, nausea, and loss of appetite.

Gastric cancer is typically diagnosed through a combination of imaging tests and biopsies. Treatment for gastric cancer depends on the stage and location of the cancer, but may include surgery, radiation therapy, chemotherapy, or a combination of these treatments.

Head and neck cancer

Head and neck cancer refers to a group of cancers that occur in the mouth, throat, nose, sinuses, and salivary glands. These cancers are often classified by the type of cell that is affected, such as squamous cell carcinoma or adenocarcinoma.

Risk factors for head and neck cancer include:

- Tobacco use: Smoking or using other tobacco products can increase the risk of head and neck cancer.

- Alcohol consumption: Heavy alcohol consumption over a prolonged period can increase the risk of head and neck cancer.

- Human papillomavirus (HPV) infection: Certain strains of HPV can increase the risk of head and neck cancer, particularly cancers of the oropharynx (the middle part of the throat).

- Exposure to certain chemicals: Exposure to certain chemicals, such as asbestos or wood dust, can increase the risk of head and neck cancer.

Symptoms of head and neck cancer may include a lump or sore that does not heal, persistent sore throat, difficulty swallowing, and changes in voice or speech.

Head and neck cancer is typically diagnosed through a combination of imaging tests and biopsies. Treatment for head and neck cancer depends on the stage and location of the cancer, but may include surgery, radiation therapy, chemotherapy, or a combination of these treatments.

Kidney (renal) cancer

Kidney (renal) cancer is a type of cancer that occurs in the cells of the kidney. There are several types of kidney cancer, including renal cell carcinoma and transitional cell carcinoma.

Risk factors for kidney cancer include:

- Smoking: Smoking cigarettes or cigars can increase the risk of kidney cancer.

- Obesity: Being overweight or obese can increase the risk of kidney cancer.

- High blood pressure: High blood pressure can increase the risk of kidney cancer.

- Family history: People with a family history of kidney cancer are at an increased risk of developing the disease.

Symptoms of kidney cancer may include blood in the urine, back pain, fatigue, and unexplained weight loss.

Kidney cancer is typically diagnosed through imaging tests and biopsies. Treatment for kidney cancer depends on the stage and location of the cancer, but may include surgery, radiation therapy, chemotherapy, or a combination of these treatments.

Leukemia

Leukemia is a type of cancer that affects the blood and bone marrow, where blood cells are produced. Leukemia is characterized by the production of abnormal white blood cells, which interfere with the production of normal blood cells.

Risk factors for leukemia include:

- Exposure to radiation: Exposure to high levels of radiation can increase the risk of leukemia.

- Exposure to chemicals: Exposure to certain chemicals, such as benzene, can increase the risk of leukemia.

- Genetic factors: Some types of leukemia may be linked to inherited genetic mutations.

- Immune system disorders: People with certain immune system disorders, such as Down syndrome, may be at an increased risk of developing leukemia.

Symptoms of leukemia may include fatigue, fever, easy bruising or bleeding, frequent infections, and bone pain.

Leukemia is typically diagnosed through blood tests and bone marrow biopsies. Treatment for leukemia depends on the type and stage of the cancer, but may include chemotherapy, radiation therapy, stem cell transplantation, or a combination of these treatments.

Liver cancer

Liver cancer is a type of cancer that occurs in the cells of the liver. There are several types of liver cancer, including hepatocellular carcinoma (HCC) and cholangiocarcinoma.

Symptoms of liver cancer may include abdominal pain, jaundice (yellowing of the skin and eyes), unexplained weight loss, and fatigue.

Liver cancer is typically diagnosed through imaging tests and biopsies. Treatment for liver cancer depends on the stage and location of the cancer, but may include surgery, radiation therapy, chemotherapy, or a combination of these treatments.

Lung cancer

Lung cancer is a type of cancer that begins in the cells of the lungs. It is the leading cause of cancer-related deaths worldwide.

Risk factors for lung cancer include:

- Smoking: Cigarette smoking is the leading cause of lung cancer, and smokers
  are at a much higher risk than non-smokers.

- Exposure to secondhand smoke: Exposure to secondhand smoke can also
  increase the risk of lung cancer.

- Exposure to radon: Radon is a naturally occurring gas that can build up in
  homes and other buildings. Long-term exposure to high levels of radon can
  increase the risk of lung cancer.

- Exposure to certain chemicals: Exposure to certain chemicals, such as
  asbestos, arsenic, and diesel exhaust, can increase the risk of lung cancer.

Symptoms of lung cancer may include coughing (including coughing up blood),
shortness of breath, chest pain, hoarseness, and unexplained weight loss.

Lung cancer is typically diagnosed through imaging tests and biopsies.
Treatment for lung cancer depends on the stage and location of the cancer, but
may include surgery, radiation therapy, chemotherapy, targeted therapy, or a
combination of these treatments.

Lymphoma

Lymphoma is a type of cancer that affects the lymphatic system, which is a part
of the immune system that helps fight infection and disease. There are two main
types of lymphoma: Hodgkin lymphoma and non-Hodgkin lymphoma.

Risk factors for lymphoma include:

- Age: Lymphoma can occur at any age, but it is more common in people over the
  age of 60.

- Weakened immune system: People with weakened immune systems, such as
  those with HIV or who have had an organ transplant, are at an increased risk
  of developing lymphoma.

- Family history: Having a close relative with lymphoma may increase the risk
  of developing the disease.

- Exposure to certain chemicals: Exposure to certain chemicals, such as
  herbicides and pesticides, has been linked to an increased risk of lymphoma.

Symptoms of lymphoma may include swollen lymph nodes, fever, night sweats,
weight loss, fatigue, and unexplained itching.

Lymphoma is typically diagnosed through a biopsy of an enlarged lymph node or
other affected tissue. Treatment for lymphoma depends on the type and stage of
the disease, but may include chemotherapy, radiation therapy, targeted therapy,
or a combination of these treatments.

Melanoma

Melanoma is a type of skin cancer that develops in the cells that produce
pigment (color) in the skin. It can occur anywhere on the body, but is most
commonly found on the legs, arms, and face.

Risk factors for melanoma include:

- Sun exposure: Exposure to ultraviolet (UV) radiation from the sun or tanning
  beds is a major risk factor for melanoma.

- Fair skin: People with fair skin, light hair, and light-colored eyes are at an
  increased risk of melanoma, as they have less natural protection against UV
  radiation.

- Family history: Having a close relative with melanoma may increase the risk of
  developing the disease.

- Weakened immune system: People with weakened immune systems, such as
  those with HIV or who have had an organ transplant, are at an increased risk
  of developing melanoma.

Symptoms of melanoma may include changes in the size, shape, or color of a
mole or other skin lesion, as well as new or unusual growths on the skin.
Melanoma may also cause itching, bleeding, or crusting of the affected area.

Melanoma is typically diagnosed through a biopsy of the affected skin or tissue.
Treatment for melanoma depends on the stage of the disease and may include

surgery, radiation therapy, chemotherapy, targeted therapy, or a combination of these treatments.

Ovarian cancer

Ovarian cancer is a type of cancer that begins in the ovaries, which are the female reproductive organs that produce eggs. It often goes undetected until it has spread to other parts of the body, which can make it more difficult to treat.

Risk factors for ovarian cancer include:

- Age: Ovarian cancer is more common in women over the age of 50.

- Family history: Women with a family history of ovarian cancer, breast cancer, or certain genetic mutations (such as BRCA1 or BRCA2) are at an increased risk of developing ovarian cancer.

- Personal history: Women who have had breast cancer, endometriosis, or certain types of infertility treatment may be at an increased risk of ovarian cancer.

- Hormone therapy: Long-term use of hormone replacement therapy (HRT) may increase the risk of ovarian cancer.

Symptoms of ovarian cancer may include bloating, pelvic or abdominal pain, difficulty eating or feeling full quickly, and urinary symptoms such as urgency or frequency. However, these symptoms can be vague and may be attributed to other conditions, which can make ovarian cancer difficult to diagnose.

There are different types of ovarian cancer, including epithelial ovarian cancer (which is the most common type), germ cell tumors, and stromal tumors. Treatment for ovarian cancer typically involves surgery to remove the tumor and surrounding tissue, followed by chemotherapy. The stage of the cancer and other factors, such as the woman's age and overall health, will determine the most appropriate treatment plan.

Pancreatic cancer

Pancreatic cancer is a type of cancer that begins in the pancreas, which is an organ located behind the stomach that produces digestive enzymes and hormones such as insulin.

Risk factors for pancreatic cancer include:

- Age: Pancreatic cancer is more common in people over the age of 60.

- Smoking: Cigarette smoking is the most important modifiable risk factor for pancreatic cancer. People who smoke cigarettes are two to three times more likely to develop pancreatic cancer compared to those who have never smoked.

- Family history: Individuals with a family history of pancreatic cancer or certain genetic syndromes (such as Lynch syndrome or hereditary breast and ovarian cancer syndrome) are at an increased risk of developing pancreatic cancer.

- Chronic pancreatitis: Long-term inflammation of the pancreas, which can be caused by heavy alcohol use or other factors, may increase the risk of pancreatic cancer.

Symptoms of pancreatic cancer may include abdominal pain, weight loss, jaundice (yellowing of the skin and eyes), and digestive problems such as nausea and vomiting. However, these symptoms can be vague and may be attributed to other conditions, which can make pancreatic cancer difficult to diagnose.

Pancreatic cancer is often aggressive and difficult to treat. Treatment may involve surgery, radiation therapy, chemotherapy, or a combination of these approaches, depending on the stage of the cancer and other factors.

Prostate cancer

Prostate cancer is a type of cancer that develops in the prostate gland, which is a small gland located between the bladder and the penis in men. The prostate gland produces fluid that nourishes and transports sperm.

Risk factors for prostate cancer include:

- Age: Prostate cancer is rare in men under 50 years of age, but the risk
  increases with age. Most cases of prostate cancer are diagnosed in men over
  the age of 65.

- Family history: Men with a family history of prostate cancer (especially if a
  close relative, such as a father or brother, has had the disease) are at an
  increased risk of developing prostate cancer themselves.

- Race: African American men and men of African descent have a higher risk of
  developing prostate cancer compared to men of other races.

- Diet: Studies suggest that diets high in red meat, dairy products, and calcium
  may increase the risk of developing prostate cancer, while diets high in fruits,
  vegetables, and certain types of fat (such as omega-3 fatty acids) may help
  reduce the risk.

Symptoms of prostate cancer may include urinary problems (such as a weak or
interrupted urine flow or frequent urination), difficulty getting or maintaining
an erection, or blood in the urine or semen. However, early-stage prostate cancer
may not cause any symptoms at all, which is why regular prostate cancer
screening (using a blood test called the prostate-specific antigen, or PSA, test) is
recommended for men at average risk starting at age 50 (or earlier for men at
higher risk).

Prostate cancer is often slow-growing and may not require treatment right
away, especially in older men or men with other health conditions. Treatment
options for prostate cancer may include surgery, radiation therapy, hormonal
therapy, or a combination of these approaches, depending on the stage of the
cancer and other factors.

Sarcoma (soft tissue and bone tumors)

Sarcomas are cancers that arise from the connective tissues in the body, such as
bone, muscle, fat, and cartilage. Sarcomas are relatively rare and account for
less than 1% of all adult cancers, but they can affect people of all ages.

There are two main types of sarcoma: soft tissue sarcoma and bone sarcoma. Soft tissue sarcomas can occur anywhere in the body, but most commonly develop in the arms, legs, chest, or abdomen. Bone sarcomas typically develop in the long bones of the arms and legs, but can also occur in other bones.

The risk factors for sarcoma are not well understood, but certain genetic conditions such as neurofibromatosis type 1, Li-Fraumeni syndrome, and retinoblastoma have been linked to an increased risk of developing sarcoma. Exposure to radiation therapy and certain chemicals may also increase the risk of sarcoma.

The unique characteristics of sarcoma depend on the specific type and location of the cancer. Symptoms may include a lump or swelling in the affected area, pain, and/or restricted movement. Diagnosis is typically made through a combination of imaging tests and biopsy.

Skin cancer

Skin cancer is the most common type of cancer, with millions of cases diagnosed each year worldwide. There are several types of skin cancer, but the most common are basal cell carcinoma, squamous cell carcinoma, and melanoma.

Basal cell carcinoma and squamous cell carcinoma are the most common types of skin cancer, and they typically develop on sun-exposed areas of the body such as the face, neck, arms, and hands. These types of skin cancer are often caused by exposure to ultraviolet (UV) radiation from the sun or from tanning beds. Other risk factors for these types of skin cancer include fair skin, a history of sunburns, a weakened immune system, and exposure to certain chemicals.

Melanoma is a less common but more dangerous type of skin cancer that can develop anywhere on the body, even in areas not exposed to the sun. Melanoma is also caused by UV radiation exposure, but it can also be caused by genetic factors. People with fair skin, a history of sunburns, a family history of melanoma, and a large number of moles are at higher risk of developing melanoma.

The unique characteristics of skin cancer depend on the specific type of cancer. Basal cell carcinoma and squamous cell carcinoma typically appear as a pink, red, or white bump or patch on the skin that may bleed or scab over. Melanoma typically appears as an irregularly shaped mole or dark spot on the skin that

may change in size, shape, or color over time. Diagnosis is typically made
through a skin biopsy.

Testicular cancer

Testicular cancer is a type of cancer that develops in the testicles, which are the
male reproductive glands located in the scrotum. Testicular cancer is relatively
rare, but it is the most common type of cancer in men between the ages of 15
and 35. The exact cause of testicular cancer is not known, but there are several
risk factors that increase the chances of developing this cancer.

Risk factors for testicular cancer include:

- Age: Testicular cancer is most common in young men between the ages of 15
  and 35.

- Cryptorchidism: This is a condition where one or both testicles fail to descend
  into the scrotum during fetal development. Men with cryptorchidism are at
  increased risk of developing testicular cancer.

- Family history: Men with a family history of testicular cancer are at increased
  risk of developing the disease.

- HIV infection: Men with HIV infection are at increased risk of developing
  testicular cancer.

- Race/ethnicity: Testicular cancer is more common in white men than in men of
  other races/ethnicities.

The most common symptom of testicular cancer is a painless lump or swelling in
one of the testicles. Other symptoms may include a feeling of heaviness in the
scrotum, pain or discomfort in the testicle or scrotum, and a dull ache in the
lower abdomen or groin. Treatment for testicular cancer usually involves
surgery to remove the affected testicle, followed by radiation therapy or
chemotherapy if the cancer has spread to other parts of the body. In most cases,
testicular cancer can be cured if it is detected and treated early.

Thyroid cancer

Thyroid cancer develops in the thyroid gland, which is located in the neck and produces hormones that regulate metabolism. It is one of the less common types of cancer, but its incidence has been increasing in recent years.

There are several types of thyroid cancer, including:

- Papillary thyroid cancer: This is the most common type of thyroid cancer and accounts for about 80% of all cases. It tends to grow slowly and is generally considered to be a less aggressive type of cancer.

- Follicular thyroid cancer: This type accounts for about 10-15% of thyroid cancers and tends to occur in older adults. It may spread to nearby lymph nodes or to other parts of the body.

- Medullary thyroid cancer: This rare type of thyroid cancer develops in cells that produce the hormone calcitonin. It can run in families and is sometimes associated with other endocrine disorders.

- Anaplastic thyroid cancer: This is a rare and aggressive type of thyroid cancer that accounts for about 2% of cases.

Risk factors for thyroid cancer include:

- Being female

- Age (most common in people over age 40)

- Exposure to radiation, particularly in childhood

- Family history of thyroid cancer or other endocrine disorders such as multiple endocrine neoplasia syndrome

Symptoms of thyroid cancer may include a lump or swelling in the neck, difficulty breathing or swallowing, hoarseness, and pain in the throat or neck.

Uterine cancer

Uterine cancer, also known as endometrial cancer, begins in the lining of the uterus (endometrium). It is the fourth most common cancer among women worldwide, with over 400,000 new cases diagnosed annually.

Risk factors for uterine cancer include:

- Age: Uterine cancer is most commonly diagnosed in women who have gone through menopause, with the average age at diagnosis being 60 years old.

- Hormone imbalances: High levels of estrogen, such as those associated with obesity, estrogen therapy, or a late onset of menopause, can increase the risk of uterine cancer.

- Family history: Women who have a family history of uterine, ovarian, or colorectal cancer may have a higher risk of developing uterine cancer.

- Genetics: Some inherited genetic mutations, such as Lynch syndrome, increase the risk of uterine cancer.

- Race: African-American women have a higher incidence of uterine cancer compared to women of other races.

- Other medical conditions: Women with a history of diabetes, polycystic ovary syndrome (PCOS), or endometrial hyperplasia (a condition in which the uterine lining becomes too thick) may have an increased risk of uterine cancer.

Symptoms of uterine cancer may include abnormal vaginal bleeding, including bleeding after menopause or between periods, pelvic pain, and abnormal discharge.

Vulvar cancer

Vulvar cancer is a rare type of cancer that starts in the outer surface of the female genitalia, called the vulva. The vulva includes the clitoris, labia minora and labia majora, vaginal opening and Bartholin's glands. Like other cancers, vulvar cancer can develop when the cells in the vulva start growing uncontrollably.

There are two main types of vulvar cancer:

Squamous cell carcinoma: This is the most common type of vulvar cancer, accounting for about 90% of all cases. Squamous cell carcinoma develops in the thin, flat cells that line the surface of the vulva.

Melanoma: This is a less common type of vulvar cancer, accounting for about 4% of all cases. It develops in the pigment-producing cells called melanocytes.

Risk factors for vulvar cancer include:

- Age: Most cases of vulvar cancer are diagnosed in women over the age of 50.

- HPV infection: Human papillomavirus (HPV) is a sexually transmitted infection that can increase the risk of vulvar cancer.

- Smoking: Smoking can increase the risk of developing vulvar cancer.

- Vulvar intraepithelial neoplasia (VIN): VIN is a precancerous condition that can increase the risk of developing vulvar cancer.

- Lichen sclerosus: This is a chronic inflammatory skin condition that can increase the risk of developing vulvar cancer.

Symptoms of vulvar cancer may include persistent itching or burning sensation in the vulva , pain or tenderness in the vulva. ,changes in the color or thickness of the skin in the vulva, a lump or growth on the vulva, bleeding or discharge not related to menstruation or pain during sexual intercourse.

- # **Diagnosis**

Diagnostic testing for cancer typically involves a combination of procedures, including imaging tests, blood tests, and tissue biopsies.

Imaging tests: Imaging tests are used to create detailed pictures of the inside of the body. Common imaging tests used to diagnose cancer include X-rays, computed tomography (CT) scans, magnetic resonance imaging (MRI) scans, ultrasound, and positron emission tomography (PET) scans.

Blood tests: Blood tests can be used to detect certain substances in the blood that may indicate the presence of cancer. For example, elevated levels of certain proteins, called tumor markers, may indicate the presence of certain types of cancer.

Biopsies:

Biopsies involve removing a small sample of tissue from the affected area and examining it under a microscope to look for cancer cells. Biopsies can be performed in a number of ways, depending on the location of the tumor. For example, a biopsy may be performed using a needle or during a surgical procedure.

In addition to these diagnostic tests, doctors may also use other procedures to help diagnose cancer. For example, endoscopy may be used to examine the inside of the digestive tract or other organs, and bone marrow aspiration and biopsy may be used to look for cancer in the bone marrow.

Overall, the diagnostic process for cancer can be complex and may involve a variety of different tests and procedures. If cancer is suspected, it is important to consult with a qualified healthcare provider who can help guide you through the diagnostic process and determine the most appropriate course of treatment.

Treatment of cancer

The treatment of cancer depends on various factors, such as the type and stage of cancer, the patient's overall health, and the potential side effects of the treatment. There are several different types of cancer treatment, including:

Surgery:

Surgery is one of the main treatments for cancer. It involves the physical removal of cancerous tissue from the body. Depending on the location and size of the tumor, surgery can be a curative or palliative treatment option.

There are several different types of surgical procedures that may be used to treat cancer, including:

Curative surgery:

This type of surgery aims to remove the entire tumor along with some surrounding healthy tissue. The goal is to remove all of the cancerous cells so that the cancer cannot come back.

Preventive surgery:

This type of surgery is used to remove tissue that is at high risk of developing cancer. For example, a woman with a strong family history of breast cancer may choose to have a preventive mastectomy (removal of both breasts) to reduce her risk of developing breast cancer.

Palliative surgery:

This type of surgery is used to relieve symptoms or improve quality of life for patients with advanced cancer. For example, surgery may be used to remove a tumor that is causing pain or to open up a blocked airway.

Reconstructive surgery:

This type of surgery is often performed after curative or preventive surgery to rebuild or reshape an area of the body that has been affected by the surgery. For example, breast reconstruction may be performed after a mastectomy. Surgery may be performed alone or in combination with other treatments such as chemotherapy or radiation therapy. The type of surgery used will depend on several factors, including the type and stage of cancer, the patient's overall health, and the goals of treatment.

Radiation therapy:

Radiation therapy is another treatment option for cancer patients. It involves the use of high-energy radiation to kill cancer cells or prevent them from multiplying. Radiation therapy can be used alone or in combination with other treatments like surgery or chemotherapy.

There are two main types of radiation therapy: external beam radiation therapy and internal radiation therapy. External beam radiation therapy involves the use of a machine that directs radiation beams to the affected area from outside the body. Internal radiation therapy, also known as brachytherapy, involves the placement of a radioactive source directly into or near the tumor.

Radiation therapy can cause side effects, including fatigue, skin irritation, and nausea. The side effects vary depending on the location of the treatment and the dose of radiation. Most side effects are temporary and can be managed with medications or other treatments.

Radiation therapy is carefully planned and monitored by a team of radiation oncologists, medical physicists, and radiation therapists. The treatment plan is personalized to each patient, taking into account the type and stage of cancer, the location of the tumor, and the patient's overall health.

Overall, radiation therapy can be an effective treatment option for many types of cancer. It may be used as the primary treatment or in combination with other treatments to help control or eliminate the cancer.

Chemotherapy:

Chemotherapy is a cancer treatment that uses drugs to kill cancer cells or prevent them from growing and dividing. Chemotherapy drugs work by targeting fast-growing cancer cells, but they can also affect healthy cells that divide rapidly, such as those in the bone marrow, hair follicles, and digestive tract. This can cause side effects, such as hair loss, nausea, and an increased risk of infection.

Chemotherapy may be given in different forms, including pills, injections, or infusion into a vein or artery. The choice of chemotherapy drugs, the dosage, and the duration of treatment depend on the type and stage of cancer, the patient's overall health, and other factors.

Chemotherapy can be used in different settings:

- Adjuvant chemotherapy: Given after surgery or radiation therapy to kill any remaining cancer cells and reduce the risk of recurrence.

- Neoadjuvant chemotherapy: Given before surgery to shrink the tumor and make it easier to remove.

- Palliative chemotherapy: Given to relieve symptoms and improve quality of life in patients with advanced cancer.

Chemotherapy can also be used in combination with other cancer treatments, such as surgery, radiation therapy, or targeted therapy. The goal of combination therapy is to improve treatment outcomes and reduce the risk of cancer recurrence.

Although chemotherapy can be an effective treatment for many types of cancer, it has some limitations. Some cancer cells may be resistant to chemotherapy, and it may not be able to completely eliminate all cancer cells in some cases. Moreover, chemotherapy can cause significant side effects and impact the patient's quality of life. Therefore, the decision to undergo chemotherapy should be made after careful consideration of the potential benefits and risks, and in consultation with a cancer specialist.

Immunotherapy:

Immunotherapy is a type of cancer treatment that uses the body's own immune system to fight cancer. The immune system is the body's natural defense against disease, and it is responsible for recognizing and attacking foreign invaders such as bacteria and viruses.

Immunotherapy works by boosting or enhancing the body's immune response against cancer cells. There are several different types of immunotherapy, including:

Checkpoint inhibitors:

These drugs block certain proteins on cancer cells that help them evade the immune system. By blocking these proteins, checkpoint inhibitors allow the immune system to recognize and attack cancer cells more effectively.

CAR-T cell therapy:

This type of immunotherapy involves collecting a patient's T cells (a type of immune cell) and modifying them in a laboratory so that they can better recognize and attack cancer cells. The modified T cells are then infused back into the patient's body.

Cancer vaccines:

These vaccines are designed to stimulate the immune system to recognize and attack cancer cells. They can be made from cancer cells, parts of cancer cells, or substances that are similar to those found on cancer cells.

Immune system modulators:

These drugs work by altering the way the immune system functions. They can help stimulate the immune system to attack cancer cells or suppress the immune system to prevent it from attacking healthy cells.

Immunotherapy has shown promise in the treatment of several types of cancer, including melanoma, lung cancer, bladder cancer, and kidney cancer. However, it is not effective for everyone, and it can cause side effects, such as fatigue, fever, and skin reactions.

Targeted therapy:

Targeted therapy is a type of cancer treatment that targets specific genes, proteins, or other molecules involved in the growth and spread of cancer cells. Unlike chemotherapy, which can damage healthy cells as well as cancer cells, targeted therapy is designed to more selectively attack cancer cells while minimizing harm to healthy cells.

Targeted therapy drugs can be classified into several categories, including:

Monoclonal antibodies:

These drugs are designed to recognize and attach to specific proteins on the surface of cancer cells, making it easier for the immune system to target and destroy them.

Small-molecule drugs:

These drugs are designed to enter the cell and interfere with specific molecules or pathways that are necessary for cancer cells to grow and survive.

Hormone therapies:

These drugs are used to block the action of certain hormones that can promote the growth of certain types of cancer cells, such as breast and prostate cancer.

Signal transduction inhibitors:

These drugs target specific signaling pathways inside the cell that are involved in the growth and survival of cancer cells.

Targeted therapy is often used in combination with other treatments, such as chemotherapy or radiation therapy, to improve their effectiveness. The side effects of targeted therapy vary depending on the drug used, but can include skin rashes, nausea, diarrhea, fatigue, and high blood pressure.

Overall, targeted therapy has shown promise in treating certain types of cancer, including breast, lung, and colorectal cancer. However, like any cancer treatment, it is not without risks and potential side effects, and its effectiveness can vary depending on the individual and the specific type of cancer being treated.

Hormone therapy:

Hormone therapy is a type of cancer treatment that is used to slow down or stop the growth of certain types of cancer that are hormone-sensitive. Hormone-sensitive cancers, such as breast and prostate cancer, grow in response to the hormones estrogen or testosterone. Hormone therapy works by either blocking the production of these hormones or blocking their effect on cancer cells.

The goal of hormone therapy is to either reduce the level of hormones in the body or to block the effect of hormones on cancer cells.
This can be done in a number of ways, including:

Medications:

Hormone therapy medications are designed to block the production or action of hormones in the body. For example, drugs such as tamoxifen and aromatase inhibitors are used to treat breast cancer by blocking the effects of estrogen.

Surgery:

In some cases, surgery may be used to remove the organs that produce hormones, such as the ovaries in women or the testicles in men.

Radiation therapy:

Radiation therapy can be used to destroy or damage hormone-producing cells, reducing the amount of hormones in the body.

Hormone therapy is often used in combination with other cancer treatments, such as chemotherapy or radiation therapy, to increase their effectiveness. The specific type of hormone therapy used will depend on the type and stage of cancer being treated, as well as the patient's overall health and other factors. Hormone therapy may also have side effects, such as hot flashes, fatigue, and decreased libido.

The choice of treatment will depend on the specific type and stage of cancer, as well as the patient's overall health and preferences. In some cases, a combination of treatments may be used to achieve the best possible outcome. It's important to note that not all treatments are effective for all types of cancer, and some may have significant side effects. Your doctor will work with you to determine the best course of treatment for your specific situation.

Chapter 2: Diet and Nutrition

Diet and nutrition play a critical role in our overall health, including the prevention and management of various diseases, including cancer. A balanced and nutritious diet provides the body with the necessary nutrients to maintain healthy cells, tissues, and organs. However, there are certain dietary factors and habits that have been linked to an increased risk of developing cancer. Additionally, for those who have already been diagnosed with cancer, maintaining a healthy diet and appropriate nutrition can help manage symptoms, improve treatment outcomes, and reduce the risk of cancer recurrence. In this chapter, we will explore the impact of diet and nutrition on cancer risk and prevention, as well as the role of diet in cancer treatment and management. We will also discuss specific dietary recommendations and guidelines for those living with cancer.

The importance of a healthy diet

A healthy diet is important for maintaining overall health and preventing chronic diseases such as obesity, heart disease, diabetes, and certain types of cancer. A balanced and nutritious diet provides the body with essential nutrients, vitamins, and minerals necessary for optimal functioning of various organs and systems.

Eating a variety of fruits, vegetables, whole grains, lean proteins, and healthy fats can improve cardiovascular health, promote healthy digestion, and support immune function. Additionally, a healthy diet can help regulate blood sugar levels, improve mental health and cognitive function, and maintain a healthy weight.
On the other hand, consuming a diet high in saturated and trans fats, added sugars, and processed foods can increase the risk of chronic diseases and lead to negative health outcomes.

It's important to note that a healthy diet is not just about the types of foods we eat, but also the portion sizes and frequency of meals. Overeating, consuming large portions, and eating too frequently can lead to weight gain and other negative health effects.

Overall, a healthy diet plays a crucial role in maintaining optimal health and reducing the risk of chronic diseases.

Foods to eat and avoid for cancer prevention

Eating a healthy and balanced diet can play an important role in preventing cancer. Here are some foods to eat and avoid for cancer prevention:

Foods to eat:

Fruits and vegetables:

Fruits and vegetables are an essential part of a healthy diet and are known for their cancer-fighting properties. They are packed with vitamins, minerals, antioxidants, and fiber, which can help protect cells from damage and reduce the risk of cancer.

Some specific fruits and vegetables that have been shown to have cancer-fighting properties include:

- Berries: Berries, such as blueberries, strawberries, and raspberries, are rich in antioxidants and have been found to reduce inflammation and inhibit the growth of cancer cells.

- Cruciferous vegetables: Vegetables like broccoli, cauliflower, and kale contain compounds that can help protect against cancer. They are rich in vitamins, fiber, and antioxidants that can help reduce inflammation and prevent damage to cells.

- Tomatoes: Tomatoes contain lycopene, a powerful antioxidant that has been linked to a reduced risk of several types of cancer, including prostate cancer.

- Citrus fruits: Citrus fruits like oranges, grapefruits, and lemons are rich in vitamin C, which can help protect cells from damage and boost the immune system.

- Leafy greens: Leafy greens such as spinach, kale, and collard greens are rich in vitamins, minerals, and antioxidants that can help protect against cancer.

In terms of foods to avoid for cancer prevention, it is recommended to limit processed and red meats, as well as sugary and high-fat foods. Consuming too much of these foods has been linked to an increased risk of several types of cancer. It is also important to limit alcohol consumption, as excessive drinking has been linked to an increased risk of certain types of cancer.

Whole grains:

Whole grains are an important part of a healthy diet for cancer prevention. Unlike refined grains, which have been processed to remove the bran and germ, whole grains contain all parts of the grain, including the fiber-rich bran and nutrient-dense germ. This means that whole grains are a good source of fiber, vitamins, and minerals.

Eating whole grains has been linked to a reduced risk of several types of cancer, including colorectal cancer. The fiber in whole grains helps to promote regular bowel movements and reduce the amount of time that potentially harmful substances are in contact with the intestinal lining. Additionally, the germ and bran in whole grains contain antioxidants that can help to reduce inflammation and protect against cellular damage.

Examples of whole grains include:

- Brown rice
- Quinoa
- Whole wheat
- Oats
- Barley
- Buckwheat
- Millet
- Rye
- Corn

When selecting whole grain products, it's important to read the ingredient list to ensure that the product is truly made with whole grains. Look for products that list a whole grain as the first ingredient, and avoid products that contain refined grains or added sugars. Additionally, it's important to be mindful of portion sizes, as even healthy foods can contribute to weight gain and other health issues if consumed in excess.

Lean proteins:

Lean proteins are an important part of a healthy diet and can provide many benefits for cancer prevention. Lean proteins are low in saturated fat and are an excellent source of nutrients such as iron, zinc, and vitamin B12.
Some examples of lean proteins include:

- Fish: Fatty fish such as salmon, tuna, and mackerel are rich in omega-3 fatty acids, which have been shown to have anti-inflammatory properties that may help reduce the risk of cancer.

- Poultry: Chicken and turkey are lean sources of protein that can be a healthy addition to your diet. Be sure to remove the skin, which is high in saturated fat.

- Beans and legumes: These are a great vegetarian source of protein and can provide many other nutrients such as fiber, folate, and potassium.

- Nuts and seeds: These are another great vegetarian source of protein and are also rich in healthy fats, fiber, and antioxidants.

It's important to note that while lean proteins can be a healthy addition to your diet, it's also important to limit your intake of processed and red meats. Studies have shown that a diet high in these meats may increase the risk of certain types of cancer, particularly colorectal cancer.

Healthy fats:

Healthy fats, also known as unsaturated fats, are an important part of a balanced diet. These fats can help reduce inflammation in the body, which can lower the risk of developing certain types of cancer, as well as other chronic conditions like heart disease and diabetes.

Sources of healthy fats include:

- Nuts and seeds (such as almonds, walnuts, chia seeds, and flaxseeds)
- Avocados
- Olive oil
- Canola oil
- Fatty fish (such as salmon, tuna, and trout)
- Soybeans and soy products (such as tofu and edamame)

It's important to note that while healthy fats can be beneficial, they are still high in calories. As with any food, it's important to consume them in moderation and be mindful of portion sizes. Additionally, it's important to limit or avoid unhealthy fats, such as saturated and trans fats, which can increase the risk of certain cancers and other health problems. Sources of unhealthy fats include fried foods, processed snacks, and fatty meats.

Foods to avoid:

Processed and packaged foods:

Processed and packaged foods are often high in calories, unhealthy fats, salt, and sugar. These types of foods include fast food, chips, crackers, cookies, sugary drinks, and processed meats. They are often low in nutrients and high in unhealthy additives, such as preservatives, artificial colors and flavors, and high-fructose corn syrup.

Consuming high amounts of processed and packaged foods has been linked to an increased risk of developing various types of cancer, such as colorectal cancer, breast cancer, and pancreatic cancer. These foods may also contribute to obesity, which is a risk factor for several types of cancer.

It is important to limit the consumption of processed and packaged foods in a healthy diet. Instead, focus on consuming fresh, whole foods that are high in nutrients and low in unhealthy additives. This includes fruits, vegetables, whole grains, lean proteins, and healthy fats. When purchasing packaged foods, read labels carefully and look for products that are low in sugar, salt, and unhealthy fats.

Sugary drinks:

Sugary drinks refer to any beverage that contains added sugar, such as soda, fruit drinks, sports drinks, and sweetened coffee or tea. These drinks can contribute to weight gain and increase the risk of developing type 2 diabetes, heart disease, and certain cancers, including breast, colon, and pancreatic cancer.

Several studies have shown that regularly consuming sugary drinks can also increase the risk of developing certain types of cancer, such as bladder and kidney cancer. This is believed to be due to the high levels of sugar in these drinks, which can lead to insulin resistance and inflammation, both of which are thought to contribute to cancer development.

To reduce the risk of cancer and improve overall health, it is recommended to limit or avoid sugary drinks and opt for healthier alternatives such as water, unsweetened tea or coffee, or low-fat milk. For those who enjoy a sweetened beverage, using natural sweeteners such as honey or maple syrup in moderation can be a better option than highly processed sugars found in sugary drinks.

Alcohol:

Alcohol consumption is a known risk factor for several types of cancer, including liver, breast, and colorectal cancer. The risk of cancer increases with the amount of alcohol consumed.

When alcohol is consumed, the body breaks it down into acetaldehyde, a toxic chemical that can damage DNA and proteins in cells. This damage can lead to the development of cancer over time.

The American Cancer Society recommends limiting alcohol consumption to no more than one drink per day for women and two drinks per day for men. A standard drink is defined as 12 ounces of beer, 5 ounces of wine, or 1.5 ounces of distilled spirits.

It is also important to note that drinking alcohol can have other negative health effects beyond the increased risk of cancer, such as liver damage, high blood pressure, and increased risk of accidents and injuries. It is always best to consume alcohol in moderation, if at all, and to prioritize other healthy behaviors such as regular exercise and a balanced diet.

High-fat meats:

High-fat meats, such as red meat (beef, pork, and lamb) and processed meats (hot dogs, bacon, and deli meats), have been linked to an increased risk of certain types of cancer, particularly colorectal cancer. The World Health Organization has classified processed meats as a Group 1 carcinogen, meaning that there is sufficient evidence to indicate that they can cause cancer in humans.

Consuming high amounts of red and processed meats may increase the risk of cancer due to several reasons. Firstly, these meats are high in saturated fat, which has been linked to an increased risk of cancer. Additionally, they contain heme iron, a type of iron that can damage cells and promote the growth of cancer cells. Finally, when meats are cooked at high temperatures (such as grilling or frying), they can form carcinogenic compounds such as polycyclic aromatic hydrocarbons (PAHs) and heterocyclic amines (HCAs).

To reduce the risk of cancer, it is recommended to limit the consumption of red and processed meats. The American Cancer Society suggests consuming no more than three servings of red meat per week and avoiding processed meats altogether. Choosing leaner cuts of meat, such as skinless chicken or turkey, fish, or plant-based protein sources like beans and legumes, can also help to reduce the amount of saturated fat in the diet.

It's important to remember that a healthy diet is just one piece of the puzzle when it comes to cancer prevention. Other lifestyle factors like regular exercise, maintaining a healthy weight, and not smoking are also important.

The role of antioxidants in cancer prevention

Antioxidants are compounds found in many foods that protect cells from damage caused by free radicals. Free radicals are unstable molecules that can damage cells and increase the risk of chronic diseases, including cancer. Antioxidants neutralize free radicals and can help prevent cellular damage.

There are many types of antioxidants, including vitamins A, C, and E, beta-carotene, selenium, and flavonoids. These nutrients can be found in a variety of fruits, vegetables, whole grains, nuts, and seeds.

Studies have shown that a diet rich in antioxidants can help reduce the risk of certain types of cancer. For example, one study found that women who consumed high levels of vitamin C had a lower risk of breast cancer than those who consumed low levels. Another study found that men who consumed high levels of selenium had a lower risk of prostate cancer than those who consumed low levels.

However, it's important to note that taking antioxidant supplements is not recommended for cancer prevention. In fact, some studies have suggested that high-dose antioxidant supplements may actually increase the risk of cancer. It's best to obtain antioxidants through a balanced diet rather than through supplements.

It's also important to note that while antioxidants can help reduce the risk of cancer, they should not be relied upon as the only means of cancer prevention. A healthy diet that includes a variety of fruits, vegetables, whole grains, and lean proteins, along with regular exercise and other healthy lifestyle choices, is the most effective way to reduce the risk of cancer.

Plant-based diets and cancer prevention

Plant-based diets have been studied for their potential role in reducing the risk of developing certain types of cancer. A plant-based diet is one that focuses on consuming mostly fruits, vegetables, whole grains, legumes, nuts, and seeds, while limiting or avoiding animal products such as meat, dairy, and eggs.

Research suggests that a plant-based diet may help reduce the risk of developing several types of cancer, including colorectal cancer, breast cancer, prostate cancer, and lung cancer. This may be due to the high levels of antioxidants, fiber, and phytochemicals found in plant-based foods, which have been shown to have cancer-fighting properties.

Additionally, plant-based diets may help reduce inflammation in the body, which has been linked to an increased risk of cancer. Studies have also found that plant-based diets may help with weight management, which can further reduce the risk of developing certain types of cancer.

It is important to note that simply following a plant-based diet does not guarantee cancer prevention, and other factors such as overall lifestyle habits and genetics also play a role. However, incorporating more plant-based foods into one's diet may offer potential benefits for reducing the risk of cancer and improving overall health.

The benefits of maintaining a healthy weight

Maintaining a healthy weight is important for overall health and can also play a role in reducing the risk of developing certain types of cancer. Excess body weight, particularly obesity, has been linked to an increased risk of several types of cancer, including breast, colon, kidney, pancreas, and endometrial cancer.

Being overweight or obese can increase the levels of certain hormones in the body, such as insulin and estrogen, which can stimulate the growth of cancer cells. In addition, excess body fat can cause chronic inflammation, which can also contribute to the development of cancer.

Maintaining a healthy weight can help to lower the levels of these hormones and reduce inflammation in the body, potentially lowering the risk of developing cancer. Even modest weight loss can have a significant impact on reducing cancer risk.

In addition to reducing cancer risk, maintaining a healthy weight can also have other health benefits, such as reducing the risk of heart disease, diabetes, and other chronic conditions. The best way to achieve and maintain a healthy weight is through a combination of a healthy diet and regular physical activity.

Chapter 3: Exercise and Physical Activity

This part will focus on the importance of exercise and physical activity in reducing the risk of cancer and promoting overall health and well-being. Regular exercise has been shown to have numerous benefits, including strengthening the immune system, reducing inflammation, improving cardiovascular health, and helping to maintain a healthy weight. Additionally, physical activity can help to decrease the risk of certain types of cancer, such as breast, colon, and endometrial cancer. This chapter will explore the different types and intensities of exercise, as well as recommendations for incorporating physical activity into daily life.

The importance of exercise for cancer prevention and overall health

Regular exercise and physical activity are essential for maintaining good health and reducing the risk of chronic diseases, including cancer. Studies have shown that physical activity can help to prevent many types of cancer, including breast, colon, endometrial, and lung cancer, as well as improve outcomes for those who have already been diagnosed with cancer.

Exercise has several benefits for cancer prevention and overall health. It helps to maintain a healthy weight, reduce inflammation, and improve immune function, all of which can help to prevent cancer. Physical activity also helps to reduce the levels of certain hormones in the body, such as estrogen and insulin, which are associated with an increased risk of cancer.

In addition to reducing the risk of cancer, exercise can also improve overall quality of life for cancer survivors. Regular exercise has been shown to reduce fatigue, improve mood, and increase overall physical function in cancer survivors.

It is important to note that the amount and type of exercise needed for cancer prevention and overall health may vary depending on individual factors such as age, fitness level, and medical history. It is recommended that adults engage in at least 150 minutes of moderate-intensity aerobic activity or 75 minutes of vigorous-intensity aerobic activity per week, along with muscle-strengthening activities at least two days per week.

In the following sections, we will discuss the different types of physical activity and how they can be incorporated into a healthy lifestyle for cancer prevention and overall health.

Types of exercise for cancer prevention

There are several types of exercises that can be beneficial for cancer prevention, including:

Aerobic exercise:

aerobic exercise, also known as cardio exercise, is a type of exercise that increases your heart rate and breathing rate. It involves continuous movement of large muscle groups, such as those in your legs, and is usually performed for a sustained period of time, such as 30 minutes or more.

Aerobic exercise has been shown to have numerous health benefits, including reducing the risk of many chronic diseases, including cancer. Regular aerobic exercise can help maintain a healthy weight, lower blood pressure, improve cholesterol levels, reduce inflammation, and boost the immune system, all of which can contribute to a reduced risk of cancer.

Examples of aerobic exercises include walking, running, cycling, swimming, dancing, and jumping rope. To achieve the maximum benefits, it is recommended to perform aerobic exercise for at least 150 minutes per week at a moderate intensity, or 75 minutes per week at a vigorous intensity.

Aerobic exercise can be particularly beneficial for those who have been diagnosed with cancer. It can improve overall fitness, help manage side effects of cancer treatment, such as fatigue and nausea, and reduce the risk of cancer recurrence. Additionally, regular exercise can help reduce stress and anxiety, which are common during cancer treatment.

Resistance training:

Resistance training, also known as strength or weight training, involves using weights, resistance bands, or body weight exercises to increase muscle strength and endurance. It is an important component of an overall exercise program for cancer prevention and management, as it can help improve body composition, increase bone density, and enhance overall physical function.

Studies have shown that resistance training can also help improve cancer-related fatigue, a common side effect of cancer and its treatments. It has also been associated with improvements in mental health, including decreased symptoms of anxiety and depression.

Resistance training should be done at least two days per week, targeting all major muscle groups. This can include exercises such as squats, lunges, push-ups, and bicep curls, among others. It is important to start with lighter weights and gradually increase resistance as strength improves.

It is also important to note that resistance training should be tailored to individual needs and abilities, especially for cancer survivors or those currently undergoing cancer treatment. A qualified exercise professional, such as a certified personal trainer or physical therapist, can help develop a safe and effective resistance training program.

Flexibility and stretching:

Flexibility and stretching exercises are also important for maintaining overall health and preventing injury during other types of exercise. These exercises help to improve range of motion, flexibility, and mobility, which can decrease the risk of muscle strain and other injuries.

Stretching exercises can be done at any time and do not require any special equipment. Some common stretching exercises include shoulder rolls, neck stretches, hamstring stretches, and calf stretches. Yoga and Pilates are also popular forms of exercise that incorporate stretching and flexibility.

It's important to note that stretching should always be done after a warm-up and never be forced to the point of pain. Additionally, it's best to work with a qualified instructor to learn proper stretching techniques and avoid any potential injuries.
- Balance and stability:
-

Balance and stability exercises are designed to improve proprioception, which is the body's ability to sense where it is in space. These exercises help improve balance, coordination, and reduce the risk of falls, particularly in older adults. For cancer survivors, balance and stability exercises can be particularly beneficial for those who have undergone treatments that affect balance, such as chemotherapy or radiation therapy to the brain.

Examples of balance and stability exercises include standing on one *leg*, heel-to-toe walking, and various yoga poses. Tai chi, a form of exercise that originated in China, has also been shown to improve balance and reduce the risk of falls.

In addition to reducing the risk of falls, balance and stability exercises can also help improve overall physical function and quality of life. They may also help reduce the risk of injuries related to physical activity. Incorporating balance and stability exercises into a well-rounded exercise routine can help cancer survivors maintain their physical function and independence.

High-intensity interval training (HIIT):

High-intensity interval training (HIIT) is a type of exercise that involves short bursts of intense exercise followed by brief periods of recovery. HIIT has gained popularity in recent years due to its effectiveness in improving cardiovascular health, increasing strength, and promoting weight loss.

Research has also suggested that HIIT may have potential benefits for cancer prevention and management. A study published in the Journal of Physiology found that HIIT was effective in reducing markers of inflammation and improving insulin sensitivity in breast cancer survivors. Another study published in the Journal of Cancer Survivorship showed that HIIT was effective in reducing fatigue and improving quality of life in prostate cancer survivors.

However, it's important to note that HIIT may not be suitable for everyone, particularly those who are new to exercise or have certain health conditions. It's important to consult with a healthcare professional before starting any new exercise regimen, including HIIT.

It's important to note that not all types of exercise may be appropriate for everyone, especially those undergoing cancer treatment or with other health conditions. It's always best to consult with a healthcare provider or certified fitness professional to determine the most appropriate exercise plan for individual needs and limitations.

How much exercise is needed for cancer prevention

The amount of exercise needed for cancer prevention and overall health depends on various factors, including age, health status, and fitness level. The American Cancer Society recommends that adults get at least 150 minutes of moderate-intensity or 75 minutes of vigorous-intensity aerobic exercise per week. This can be achieved through activities such as brisk walking, cycling, swimming, or running.

In addition to aerobic exercise, the American Cancer Society also recommends that adults engage in muscle-strengthening activities at least two days per week.

This can include resistance training, weight lifting, or bodyweight exercises such as push-ups or squats.

It's important to note that these recommendations are a general guideline, and individuals should consult with their healthcare provider before starting an exercise program. People with cancer or undergoing cancer treatment should also consult with their healthcare provider before beginning an exercise program, as certain types of exercise may not be appropriate for their condition.

It's also important to incorporate a variety of exercise types into your routine, including aerobic exercise, resistance training, flexibility, and balance/stability exercises. This can help improve overall fitness and reduce the risk of injury. Remember, any amount of physical activity is better than none, and even small amounts of exercise can have health benefits. So if you're just starting out, begin with small amounts of physical activity and gradually increase over time as you become more comfortable and confident.

Exercise and weight management

Regular exercise can play an important role in managing weight and preventing obesity, which is a significant risk factor for many types of cancer. When combined with a healthy diet, exercise can help promote weight loss and maintenance by burning calories and building lean muscle mass.

Research suggests that engaging in moderate to vigorous physical activity for at least 150 minutes per week can lead to clinically significant weight loss and improve body composition, including reducing body fat and increasing muscle mass. This can have a positive impact on cancer risk reduction, as excess body fat can lead to inflammation, hormonal imbalances, and other biological changes that increase the risk of certain cancers.

Moreover, regular exercise has been shown to help maintain weight loss over time, which is important for long-term cancer prevention. A combination of aerobic exercise and resistance training can be especially effective in building lean muscle mass and increasing metabolic rate, leading to greater calorie burn and weight loss.
In addition to weight management, exercise can also improve overall health by reducing the risk of chronic diseases such as heart disease, type 2 diabetes, and stroke. These conditions are also risk factors for certain types of cancer, and reducing their incidence through exercise and lifestyle changes can have a positive impact on cancer prevention.

Exercise and stress reduction

Exercise can be a great way to reduce stress, which is important for overall health and may also have a positive impact on cancer prevention. When you exercise, your body releases endorphins, which are natural mood boosters that can help alleviate feelings of stress and anxiety.

In addition to the release of endorphins, exercise can also help you feel more relaxed by reducing muscle tension and promoting better sleep. When you get a good night's rest, you are more likely to feel better physically and mentally, which can in turn help you better manage stress.

Regular exercise can also help you build resilience to stress. By challenging yourself physically and mentally during workouts, you can increase your ability to handle stressful situations in other areas of your life.

Incorporating regular exercise into your routine can be an effective way to manage stress and improve your overall well-being.

Chapter 4: Environmental Factors

Chapter 4 of our guide is all about environmental factors that may increase the risk of cancer. Many environmental factors such as air pollution, water pollution, exposure to radiation, and exposure to certain chemicals have been linked to cancer. In this chapter, we will explore the various environmental factors that may contribute to cancer risk, as well as ways to reduce exposure to these factors. It is important to understand the impact of the environment on cancer risk, as it can help individuals make informed decisions about their lifestyle choices and advocate for changes in their communities to promote a healthier environment.

Environmental toxins and their link to cancer

Environmental toxins are substances that are found in the environment and can potentially cause harm to human health. Some environmental toxins have been linked to an increased risk of cancer. These toxins can be found in air, water, soil, food, and consumer products.

Examples of environmental toxins include:

Carcinogens:

Carcinogens are substances that have the potential to cause cancer. These substances can be found in both natural and man-made sources, such as tobacco smoke, air pollution, pesticides, herbicides, and some chemicals used in manufacturing. When exposed to these substances, the DNA in our cells can become damaged, which can lead to the development of cancer.

Carcinogens can be classified into different categories based on the degree of evidence supporting their ability to cause cancer. Some carcinogens, like tobacco smoke and ultraviolet (UV) radiation from the sun, are considered to be well-established carcinogens, while others are still being studied to determine their potential risks.

It's important to note that not everyone exposed to carcinogens will develop cancer, as individual susceptibility can vary based on factors such as genetics, age, and overall health. However, reducing exposure to known carcinogens is an important step in reducing the risk of developing cancer.

Endocrine disruptors:

Endocrine disruptors are chemicals that can interfere with the normal function of the endocrine system, which is responsible for producing hormones that regulate many bodily functions. Exposure to endocrine disruptors can lead to a variety of health problems, including cancer. Some examples of endocrine disruptors include bisphenol-A (BPA), phthalates, and dioxins.

BPA is a chemical commonly used in plastics, such as water bottles, food containers, and toys. It has been linked to breast cancer, prostate cancer, and other health problems. Phthalates are often used in personal care products, such as perfumes, lotions, and shampoos. Exposure to phthalates has been linked to breast cancer, as well as reproductive problems in both men and women. Dioxins are a group of chemicals that are produced by burning certain types of waste, and can be found in some foods. Exposure to dioxins has been linked to a higher risk of certain types of cancer, including lymphoma and soft tissue sarcoma.

Endocrine disruptors are a growing concern, as they are found in many everyday products and can be difficult to avoid completely. However, there are steps that can be taken to reduce exposure, such as choosing products that are labeled as "BPA-free" or "phthalate-free," avoiding products with fragrances, and eating a diet that is low in animal fats, which can contain dioxins. Additionally, it is important to advocate for stronger regulations on the use of endocrine disruptors to protect public health.

Heavy metals:

Heavy metals are naturally occurring elements that can be toxic to humans in high concentrations. Some of the most well-known heavy metals that are linked to cancer include lead, cadmium, and mercury. Exposure to these metals can occur through a variety of sources, including contaminated food and water, air pollution, and industrial activities.

Lead is a heavy metal that was once commonly used in gasoline, paint, and plumbing materials. Today, it is still found in some older buildings and water pipes. High levels of lead exposure have been linked to an increased risk of several types of cancer, including brain cancer, lung cancer, and kidney cancer.

Cadmium is a heavy metal that is often found in soil, water, and food. It is used in some industrial processes, including the production of batteries and plastics. High levels of cadmium exposure have been linked to an increased risk of lung cancer, prostate cancer, and kidney cancer.

Mercury is a heavy metal that is found in certain types of fish, as well as in some industrial processes. Exposure to high levels of mercury has been linked to an increased risk of several types of cancer, including brain cancer and lung cancer.

Such as arsenic and chromium, have also been linked to an increased risk of cancer. Arsenic is found in some well water, and exposure to high levels of this metal has been linked to an increased risk of lung cancer, skin cancer, and bladder cancer. Chromium is used in some industrial processes, and exposure to high levels of this metal has been linked to an increased risk of lung cancer and stomach cancer.

Overall, iIof cancer and other health problems. This can be achieved through measures such as eating a healthy diet, avoiding contaminated water sources, and reducing exposure to industrial pollutants.

Radiation:

Radiation is a form of energy that travels in waves or particles, and can be found naturally or man-made. Exposure to high levels of radiation can cause damage to cells and DNA, which can increase the risk of cancer.

Sources of radiation can include medical procedures such as X-rays and CT scans, as well as radiation therapy for cancer treatment. Natural sources of radiation can come from radon gas in the environment, cosmic radiation from outer space, and exposure to the sun's ultraviolet (UV) radiation.

Exposure to high levels of radiation can cause acute health effects such as nausea, vomiting, and skin burns, as well as long-term health effects such as an increased risk of cancer. The risk of cancer depends on the type and amount of radiation exposure, as well as individual factors such as age and genetics.

Radiation can also be a carcinogen, which is a substance or agent that can cause cancer by altering DNA and promoting the growth of cancer cells. Some examples of radiation-induced cancers include leukemia and thyroid cancer.

To minimize exposure to radiation, individuals can take precautions such as using protective clothing and equipment when working with radiation, avoiding unnecessary medical procedures that involve radiation, and minimizing exposure to natural sources of radiation.

It's important to note that not all environmental toxins are carcinogenic or have been definitively linked to cancer. However, exposure to these toxins can still have negative effects on overall health and increase the risk of other health problems.
Reducing exposure to environmental toxins can be challenging, as they are often present in everyday products and substances.

There are steps that can be taken to reduce exposure, such as:

Quitting smoking and avoiding exposure to secondhand smoke.

Eating a diet that is low in processed and packaged foods, and high in whole foods, fruits, and vegetables.

Using non-toxic household cleaning and personal care products.

Filtering drinking water and avoiding exposure to contaminated water sources.

Minimizing exposure to radiation, such as by wearing protective gear during certain medical procedures.

Properly disposing of hazardous materials, such as batteries and electronics.

By taking these steps, individuals can reduce their exposure to environmental toxins and potentially lower their risk of cancer and other health problems.

Common environmental toxins to avoid

There are several common environmental toxins that people should try to avoid to reduce their risk of cancer. These include:

Pesticides:

Pesticides are chemicals used to control or eliminate pests such as insects, rodents, and weeds. They are commonly used in agriculture to protect crops and ensure high yields. However, pesticides can also pose a threat to human health and the environment. Exposure to pesticides has been linked to an increased risk of cancer, as well as other health problems such as respiratory issues, neurological disorders, and reproductive problems.

One of the main concerns with pesticide exposure is through the consumption of contaminated fruits and vegetables. In order to reduce exposure, it is recommended to buy organic produce whenever possible, and to thoroughly wash all produce before consumption. It is also important to follow proper handling and disposal protocols when using pesticides in and around the home.

Individuals who work with or around pesticides, such as farmers and farm workers, are at a higher risk of exposure and should take extra precautions to protect themselves. This may include using personal protective equipment, following safe handling practices, and regularly monitoring their health for any signs of exposure.

Reducing exposure to pesticides is an important step in preventing cancer and other health problems. This can be achieved through purchasing organic produce, properly washing produce, and following safe handling practices for pesticides.

Air pollution:

Air pollution is a major environmental factor that has been linked to various health issues, including cancer. Air pollution is made up of a mixture of gases, particles, and other substances that can be harmful to human health when breathed in. There are two main types of air pollution: outdoor and indoor.

Outdoor air pollution is caused by a variety of factors, including vehicle exhaust, industrial emissions, and wildfires. Exposure to outdoor air pollution has been linked to an increased risk of lung cancer, as well as other types of cancer such as bladder, breast, and stomach cancer.

Indoor air pollution can be caused by a variety of factors, including tobacco smoke, cooking fumes, and chemicals released from building materials and furnishings. Exposure to indoor air pollution has been linked to an increased risk of lung cancer, as well as other types of cancer such as leukemia and lymphoma.

To reduce your exposure to air pollution, it's important to be aware of the air quality in your area and take steps to protect yourself. This can include using air purifiers in your home, avoiding exercising outdoors during times of high pollution, and reducing your use of cars and other vehicles that contribute to outdoor pollution. Additionally, quitting smoking and avoiding exposure to secondhand smoke can help reduce your risk of lung cancer.

Household chemicals:

Household chemicals are commonly found in many everyday products used in households, including cleaning products, personal care products, and home improvement materials. These chemicals can include a variety of ingredients, such as solvents, fragrances, and preservatives, that can have harmful effects on human health and the environment.

Some common household chemicals that may have a potential link to cancer include:

- Phthalates: These are chemicals used in many personal care products and plastics, and have been shown to disrupt the endocrine system and potentially increase the risk of breast cancer.

- Bisphenol A (BPA): BPA is found in many plastic products, including water bottles and food containers, and has been linked to an increased risk of breast and prostate cancers.

- Triclosan: Triclosan is an antibacterial chemical found in some soaps and toothpaste, and has been shown to disrupt hormone function and potentially increase the risk of breast and ovarian cancers.

- Formaldehyde: This chemical is commonly used in building materials, such as insulation and pressed wood products, and has been classified as a known human carcinogen by the International Agency for Research on Cancer.

- Perfluorinated compounds (PFCs): PFCs are used in many non-stick and stain-resistant products, and have been linked to an increased risk of kidney and testicular cancers.

Reducing exposure to these household chemicals can be challenging, but there are some steps that can be taken to minimize the risk. These include using natural cleaning products, choosing products with fewer chemicals, properly ventilating indoor spaces, and properly disposing of hazardous materials.

Radon:

Radon is a naturally occurring gas that can be found in soil, rock, and water. It is formed by the decay of uranium, which is present in most soils and rocks. Radon gas is odorless, colorless, and tasteless, making it difficult to detect without testing.

Radon exposure is a significant environmental risk factor for lung cancer. When radon gas is released from the ground and enters a building, it can accumulate to high levels, particularly in confined spaces such as basements. As people breathe in the air containing radon, radioactive particles from the gas can become trapped in the lungs and damage the cells, potentially leading to lung cancer.

The best way to determine the radon levels in a home or building is to conduct a radon test. There are several types of tests available, including short-term tests that take measurements over a few days to a week, and long-term tests that take measurements over several months to a year.

If high levels of radon are detected, measures can be taken to reduce exposure. Radon mitigation systems, which involve ventilation and air exchange, can be installed to reduce the concentration of radon in the air. It is important to address high levels of radon as soon as possible to reduce the risk of developing lung cancer.

By taking steps to avoid these common environmental toxins, you can help reduce your risk of cancer and promote overall health and well-being.

Reducing exposure to environmental toxins

While it's impossible to completely avoid exposure to all environmental toxins, there are steps you can take to reduce your exposure and lower your risk of developing cancer.

Here are some tips:

- Eat organic foods: Pesticides and herbicides used in conventional farming can contaminate soil, water, and food. By choosing organic produce, you can reduce your exposure to these chemicals.

- Filter your drinking water: Tap water can contain traces of heavy metals, pesticides, and other toxins. A high-quality water filter can help remove these contaminants.

- Choose natural cleaning products: Many household cleaners contain chemicals that can be harmful to your health. Look for natural alternatives, such as vinegar and baking soda, or choose cleaners labeled as "green" or « natural."

- Be careful with cosmetics: Many personal care products, such as shampoos, lotions, and makeup, contain chemicals that can be absorbed through the skin. Look for products with natural, non-toxic ingredients.

- Avoid tobacco smoke: Tobacco smoke contains dozens of known carcinogens, and exposure to secondhand smoke can also increase your risk of cancer.

- Test your home for radon: Radon is a naturally occurring gas that can seep into homes and increase the risk of lung cancer. You can test your home for radon and take steps to reduce levels if necessary.

- Reduce exposure to air pollution: Air pollution can increase the risk of lung cancer and other health problems. Avoid exercising outdoors on high-pollution days, and consider using an air purifier in your home.

By taking these steps, you can help reduce your exposure to environmental toxins and lower your risk of developing cancer.

The importance of a clean living environment

A clean living environment is essential for maintaining good health, especially when it comes to preventing cancer. Many environmental toxins can accumulate in our homes and workplaces, putting us at risk for long-term exposure. Therefore, it's important to take steps to minimize our exposure to toxins and create a clean, healthy living environment.

One of the most effective ways to reduce exposure to environmental toxins is to eliminate or reduce the use of toxic products in the home. This includes chemical cleaning products, air fresheners, pesticides, and other household chemicals that may contain harmful ingredients. Switching to natural cleaning products, such as vinegar and baking soda, can significantly reduce exposure to toxins.

Improving indoor air quality is also important for maintaining a clean living environment. Using air purifiers and ensuring proper ventilation can help remove pollutants and improve air quality. Additionally, choosing non-toxic building materials, such as low-VOC paint, can reduce exposure to harmful chemicals in the home.

Maintaining a clean living environment also involves proper storage and disposal of household waste, such as batteries, electronics, and other hazardous materials. These materials should be stored in a secure location and disposed of properly to prevent contamination of the environment.

Creating a clean living environment involves taking steps to minimize exposure to environmental toxins and pollutants, which can help reduce the risk of cancer and other health problems.

Chapter 5: Stress Management

Chapter 5 focuses on the important topic of stress management and its impact on cancer prevention. Stress can have a significant impact on the body's immune system, making it more difficult to fight off diseases like cancer. Therefore, it is essential to learn effective stress management techniques to reduce the impact of stress on the body. This chapter will explore various techniques for managing stress, including mindfulness, meditation, and yoga, as well as other lifestyle changes that can help to reduce stress levels. By implementing these strategies, individuals can improve their overall health and reduce their risk of developing cancer.

The link between stress and cancer

Research has shown that stress can have negative effects on physical and mental health, including an increased risk for cancer. Chronic stress can lead to hormonal imbalances, immune system dysfunction, and inflammation, all of which can contribute to the development and progression of cancer.

One of the hormones that can be affected by chronic stress is cortisol, which helps regulate the immune system. Prolonged stress can lead to elevated cortisol levels, which can suppress the immune system's ability to detect and destroy cancer cells. Chronic stress can also lead to inflammation, which is a key factor in the development and progression of cancer.

In addition, stress can also lead to unhealthy coping behaviors such as smoking, overeating, and excessive alcohol consumption, all of which can increase cancer risk. It is important to note that stress alone does not cause cancer, but it can contribute to the development and progression of the disease. Therefore, managing stress is an important aspect of cancer prevention and overall health.

Techniques for managing stress

Certainly! There are a variety of techniques that can be used to manage stress, and what works best will vary depending on the individual. Some common techniques include:

Meditation and mindfulness practices:

Meditation and mindfulness practices are techniques that involve focusing one's attention on the present moment, often through deep breathing and visualization. These practices have been shown to be effective in reducing stress and promoting relaxation.

Research suggests that meditation and mindfulness practices may also have benefits for cancer patients and survivors. For example, one study found that breast cancer survivors who participated in a mindfulness-based stress reduction program experienced significant reductions in symptoms of stress, anxiety, and depression.

Meditation and mindfulness practices may also help improve quality of life and reduce symptoms such as fatigue and pain in cancer patients and survivors. Additionally, these practices may improve immune function and reduce inflammation, both of which can be important factors in cancer prevention and treatment.

There are many different forms of meditation and mindfulness practices, including guided meditations, body scans, and mindful breathing exercises. These practices can be done alone or in a group setting and can be easily incorporated into daily routines.

Exercise:

Exercise is a well-known stress-relieving activity that can help reduce the negative effects of stress on the body. Even moderate exercise can release endorphins, the body's natural "feel-good" chemicals, and improve mood. Exercise can also reduce muscle tension, increase energy levels, and promote better sleep, all of which can help reduce stress.

In addition to aerobic exercise and resistance training, activities such as yoga, Pilates, and tai chi can be effective in managing stress. These practices focus on controlled movements, deep breathing, and relaxation techniques, which can help promote a sense of calm and reduce anxiety.

It's important to note that exercise can be a powerful tool in managing stress, but it's important to start slowly and choose activities that are enjoyable and sustainable. Overexertion or pushing too hard too fast can actually increase stress levels and cause injury, so it's important to listen to your body and pace yourself.

Yoga:

Yoga is a mind-body practice that originated in ancient India and has gained popularity around the world for its ability to reduce stress, increase flexibility, and promote relaxation. It involves a combination of physical postures, breathing techniques, and meditation or relaxation.

Yoga has been found to have a number of benefits for cancer patients and survivors, including improving physical function, reducing fatigue, and enhancing quality of life. A systematic review of 24 randomized controlled trials found that yoga interventions improved physical functioning, reduced fatigue, and improved quality of life in cancer patients and survivors.

Some specific benefits of yoga for cancer patients and survivors include improved sleep, reduced stress and anxiety, improved mood, and reduced pain and discomfort. Additionally, yoga may help to improve immune function and decrease inflammation, which may be beneficial in preventing cancer and supporting the body's ability to fight cancer.

There are many different styles of yoga, and it's important to find a class or teacher that is appropriate for your level of fitness and comfort level. It's also important to talk to your healthcare provider before starting a yoga practice, especially if you have any health concerns or physical limitations.

Relaxation techniques:

Relaxation techniques are an effective way to manage stress and promote a sense of calmness and well-being.
There are several different types of relaxation techniques, including:

- Deep breathing: Deep breathing is a simple yet effective relaxation technique that involves taking slow, deep breaths from the diaphragm. This type of breathing helps to slow down the heart rate and lower blood pressure, promoting a sense of relaxation and calmness.

- Progressive muscle relaxation: Progressive muscle relaxation involves tensing and relaxing each muscle group in the body, starting from the toes and working up to the head. This technique helps to release physical tension and promote a sense of relaxation.

- Visualization: Visualization involves using mental imagery to create a sense of calmness and relaxation. This technique can involve visualizing a peaceful scene, such as a beach or a forest, or imagining oneself succeeding in a particular goal.

- Massage: Massage is a hands-on relaxation technique that involves kneading and manipulating the muscles to release tension and promote relaxation.

- Mindfulness meditation: Mindfulness meditation involves being present in the moment and focusing on the sensations of the body, breath, and surroundings. This technique helps to cultivate a sense of awareness and mindfulness, reducing stress and promoting relaxation.

Incorporating relaxation techniques into one's daily routine can help to manage stress and promote overall well-being, which in turn may help to reduce the risk of developing certain health conditions, including cancer.

Social support:

Social support is a crucial component of stress management, as it can help individuals cope with stressful situations and reduce the negative impact of stress on health. Social support can come from various sources, such as family, friends, coworkers, and support groups.

Research has shown that individuals with stronger social support networks are more likely to have better physical and mental health outcomes, including a lower risk of cancer. Social support can also provide a sense of belonging, reduce feelings of loneliness and isolation, and improve overall well-being.

Some ways to build social support include joining a support group, participating in community events, volunteering, and reaching out to friends and family for help and support. Additionally, talking to a therapist or counselor can also be a valuable resource for managing stress and building social support.

It is important to note that social support is a two-way street, and individuals can also provide support to others in their network. This can not only strengthen relationships but also improve overall well-being and sense of purpose.

Time management:

Time management is a technique that involves organizing and planning how much time you spend on different activities to achieve maximum productivity and efficiency. It can be a helpful tool in managing stress, as feeling overwhelmed and having too much to do can contribute to feelings of stress and anxiety.

Effective time management can help individuals feel more in control of their daily activities and reduce the feeling of being rushed or constantly behind schedule. By prioritizing tasks and allocating time for each one, individuals can ensure that they are completing important tasks while also making time for relaxation and self-care.

Some tips for effective time management include:

- Create a daily schedule: Plan out your day in advance, setting aside specific times for work, leisure, and self-care activities.

- Prioritize tasks: Identify the most important tasks on your to-do list and focus on completing those first.

- Minimize distractions: Limit time spent on social media or other non-essential activities that can consume time and detract from productivity.

- Take breaks: Allow yourself time to rest and recharge throughout the day. Taking breaks can help prevent burnout and improve focus.

- Be realistic: Set realistic expectations for how much can be accomplished in a day, and don't overcommit to tasks that may not be achievable.

Effective time management can be an important tool in managing stress and promoting overall well-being.

Cognitive-behavioral therapy (CBT):

Cognitive-behavioral therapy (CBT) is a type of psychotherapy that focuses on changing negative thought patterns and behaviors that contribute to stress, anxiety, and other mental health issues. CBT can help individuals identify and challenge negative thought patterns and replace them with positive and constructive ones, which can lead to better stress management and overall well-being.

In the context of cancer prevention, CBT can be particularly helpful for individuals who experience high levels of stress and anxiety related to cancer risk, diagnosis, or treatment. By learning new coping skills and thought patterns, individuals can reduce their stress levels and improve their quality of life. CBT can also be useful for managing other aspects of life that may contribute to stress, such as work or family obligations.

CBT typically involves regular sessions with a licensed therapist, who may use a variety of techniques such as cognitive restructuring, behavioral activation, and relaxation training. It may also involve homework assignments and practice exercises outside of therapy sessions to reinforce new skills and behaviors.

Overall, CBT is a valuable tool for managing stress and anxiety, and it can be particularly helpful for individuals who are at increased risk of developing cancer or who are undergoing cancer treatment.

It's important to note that managing stress is a process, and what works for one person may not work for another. It may take some experimentation to find the stress management techniques that work best for you.

Mindfulness and meditation

Mindfulness and meditation are techniques that are often used in stress management and can help individuals cultivate a sense of calm and relaxation. Mindfulness is the practice of being fully present and aware of one's thoughts, feelings, and surroundings in the present moment, without judgment. It can be practiced through various techniques such as guided meditations, breathing exercises, and body scans.

Meditation, on the other hand, is a technique that involves focusing the mind on a particular object, sound, or visualization to achieve a sense of relaxation and mental clarity. There are different types of meditation, such as mantra meditation, transcendental meditation, and mindfulness meditation.

Studies have shown that mindfulness and meditation can have a positive impact on mental and physical health. For example, mindfulness-based stress reduction (MBSR) programs have been found to be effective in reducing symptoms of anxiety, depression, and stress. Mindfulness and meditation have also been linked to improvements in immune function and reductions in inflammation, which may have implications for cancer prevention and treatment.

In addition, mindfulness and meditation can help individuals build resilience to stress, which can be particularly important for cancer patients and survivors. They can also be used as a complementary therapy alongside other cancer treatments to improve overall well-being and quality of life.

Yoga and other relaxation techniques

Yoga is a practice that combines physical postures, breathing techniques, and meditation to improve overall well-being and reduce stress. It has been shown to have numerous benefits for mental and physical health, including stress reduction, improved mood, increased flexibility, and reduced inflammation.

Other relaxation techniques include deep breathing exercises, progressive muscle relaxation, guided imagery, and massage therapy. These techniques can help reduce muscle tension, lower blood pressure, and promote relaxation and calmness. Some studies suggest that regular practice of relaxation techniques can also improve immune system function and reduce inflammation.

It's important to note that different techniques may work better for different individuals, and it may take some trial and error to find the right approach for managing stress. Additionally, it's important to incorporate these techniques into a larger stress-management plan that includes healthy lifestyle habits, social support, and, if needed, professional therapy.

Here are a few examples of relaxation techniques:

- Progressive muscle relaxation: This involves tensing and then relaxing different muscle groups in your body, usually starting from your toes and working your way up to your head. It can help reduce tension and promote relaxation.

- Visualization: This involves using your imagination to create a mental image of a peaceful or calming place, such as a beach or a forest. Focusing on this image can help you relax and reduce stress.

- Deep breathing: Taking slow, deep breaths can help calm your mind and body. Try inhaling deeply through your nose, holding your breath for a few seconds, and then exhaling slowly through your mouth.

- Guided imagery: This involves listening to a recording or a guide who leads you through a visualization or meditation, helping you relax and reduce stress.

- Yoga and tai chi: These are forms of exercise that combine movement, deep breathing, and meditation. They can help improve flexibility, reduce stress, and promote relaxation.

- Aromatherapy: This involves using essential oils or other scents to create a calming or soothing environment. Some popular scents for relaxation include lavender, chamomile, and jasmine.

Relaxation techniques may work differently for different people, so it's important to find the ones that work best for you.

Chapter 6: Cancer Screening and Early Detection

Chapter 6 of this guide is dedicated to discussing the importance of cancer screening and early detection. Cancer screening is the process of looking for cancer or pre-cancerous changes in people who have no symptoms of the disease. Early detection refers to identifying cancer at an early stage, before it has had a chance to spread and become more difficult to treat. The goal of cancer screening and early detection is to increase the chances of successful treatment and improve overall survival rates. In this chapter, we will discuss different types of cancer screening tests, the benefits and risks of screening, and recommendations for when and how often to get screened.

The importance of cancer screening

Cancer screening is the process of testing for early signs of cancer in people who have no symptoms of the disease. It is an important tool for early detection and prevention of cancer, as it can help identify cancer at an early stage when treatment is likely to be more effective.

Screening tests can help detect certain types of cancer before symptoms appear. This is important because some cancers, such as breast, cervical, and colon cancer, can be treated more successfully if detected early. In some cases, screening tests can also help prevent cancer altogether, as in the case of colon cancer screening, where the removal of polyps before they become cancerous can prevent the development of cancer.

Screening tests for cancer include mammography for breast cancer, Pap tests for cervical cancer, colonoscopy for colon cancer, and PSA testing for prostate cancer. However, it's important to note that not all screening tests are appropriate for everyone, and the decision to undergo a screening test should be made in consultation with a healthcare provider based on an individual's personal and family medical history.

Cancer screening is an important part of cancer prevention and early detection, and can help save lives by identifying cancer at an early, more treatable stage.

Recommended cancer screening guidelines

The recommended cancer screening guidelines can vary depending on a person's age, gender, family history, and other risk factors. However, there are some general guidelines that healthcare professionals typically follow.

For breast cancer screening, the American Cancer Society recommends that women at average risk start getting yearly mammograms at age 45, and then switch to getting mammograms every other year at age 55. Women may also choose to start getting mammograms earlier, starting at age 40. Additionally, clinical breast exams are recommended every 3 years for women in their 20s and 30s, and yearly for women age 40 and older.

For cervical cancer screening, the American Cancer Society recommends that women start getting Pap tests at age 21. Between the ages of 21 and 29, women should have a Pap test every 3 years. Between the ages of 30 and 65, women can either continue getting a Pap test every 3 years or switch to getting a Pap test along with an HPV test every 5 years.

For colorectal cancer screening, the American Cancer Society recommends that people at average risk start getting screened at age 45. There are several screening options available, including colonoscopy, flexible sigmoidoscopy, stool tests, and virtual colonoscopy.

It's important to note that these are just general guidelines, and individual recommendations may vary based on a person's specific health history and risk factors. It's always a good idea to discuss cancer screening options with a healthcare professional.

Early detection and its impact on cancer survival rates

Early detection plays a crucial role in improving cancer survival rates. When cancer is caught at an early stage, it is often easier to treat and has a better chance of being cured. In fact, many cancers can be cured if they are detected early and treated promptly. On the other hand, if cancer is allowed to grow and spread before it is detected, it can be much more difficult to treat and the chances of a successful outcome are greatly reduced.

The impact of early detection on cancer survival rates can be seen in the statistics. For example, the 5-year survival rate for breast cancer is over 90% if it is caught early and has not spread beyond the breast. However, if the cancer has spread to other parts of the body, the 5-year survival rate drops to around 27%.

Similarly, the 5-year survival rate for colon cancer is around 90% if it is detected at an early stage, but drops to around 14% if it has spread to other parts of the body. The same is true for other types of cancer, including lung cancer, prostate cancer, and skin cancer.

Early detection is especially important for people who are at high risk of developing certain types of cancer, such as those with a family history of the disease or those who have been exposed to environmental toxins. These individuals may need to be screened more frequently or at an earlier age than the general population.

It is important to note that cancer screening tests are not perfect and may sometimes miss cancers or lead to false positives, which can cause unnecessary anxiety and further testing. However, overall, the benefits of early detection outweigh the risks, and regular cancer screening is an important part of maintaining good health.

Types of cancer screening tests

There are several types of cancer screening tests that are recommended for different types of cancer. Here are some of the most common ones:

Mammography:

Mammography is a specific type of imaging test used to detect breast cancer. It is a low-dose X-ray that produces an image of the breast tissue. Mammograms are typically recommended for women who are over the age of 50, but may be recommended at an earlier age if there is a family history of breast cancer or other risk factors.

There are two types of mammography: screening and diagnostic. Screening mammography is used to detect breast cancer in women who have no signs or symptoms of the disease. It is typically performed every one to two years for women over the age of 50. Diagnostic mammography is used to evaluate a woman who has symptoms such as a lump or breast pain.

During a mammogram, the breast is compressed between two plates to flatten and spread out the tissue. This can be uncomfortable for some women, but it only lasts a few seconds. The images produced by the mammogram are examined by a radiologist who looks for any abnormalities or areas of concern. If a suspicious area is found, further testing such as a biopsy may be recommended.

Mammography is an important tool for detecting breast cancer early, when it is most treatable. While it is not perfect and can miss some cancers or result in false positives, it remains the gold standard for breast cancer screening. It is important for women to talk to their doctor about when and how often they should have mammograms based on their individual risk factors.

Pap test:

 A Pap test, also known as a Pap smear, is a screening test used to detect abnormal cells in the cervix that may indicate the presence of cervical cancer or precancerous conditions. The test involves collecting a sample of cells from the cervix using a small brush or spatula. The sample is then examined under a microscope for abnormalities.

The American Cancer Society recommends that women with a cervix start getting Pap tests at age 25, or earlier if they have certain risk factors such as a weakened immune system or a history of cervical cancer. Women between the ages of 25 and 65 should get a Pap test every 3 years. Women over age 65 who have had regular screenings with normal results in the past should talk to their healthcare provider about whether they still need to be screened.

It's important to note that a Pap test is not a diagnostic test for cervical cancer. If abnormal cells are detected, further testing may be needed to determine if cancer is present. In addition, a Pap test does not detect other types of gynecologic cancers, such as ovarian or uterine cancer. Women should talk to their healthcare provider about the best screening schedule for their individual needs.

Colonoscopy:

Colonoscopy is a type of cancer screening test that is used to detect abnormalities or growths in the colon or rectum, which are known as polyps. During a colonoscopy, a long, flexible tube with a camera on the end is inserted into the rectum and guided through the colon. The camera allows the doctor to view the lining of the colon and identify any abnormalities.

Colonoscopy is recommended as a screening test for colon cancer starting at age 50 for people at average risk, or earlier for those with a family history of colon cancer or other risk factors. During the procedure, if any polyps are found, they can be removed during the colonoscopy, which can help to prevent colon cancer from developing.

The preparation for a colonoscopy involves a special diet and a bowel-cleansing regimen to ensure that the colon is free of any stool or other material that could interfere with the doctor's ability to see the colon lining. The procedure itself usually takes between 30 minutes to an hour, and patients are usually given sedation to help them relax and minimize any discomfort.

In addition to detecting colon cancer, colonoscopy can also be used to diagnose other conditions, such as inflammatory bowel disease and diverticulitis. It is important to follow the recommended screening guidelines for colonoscopy, as early detection can lead to more effective treatment and better outcomes.

Prostate-specific antigen (PSA) test:

The prostate-specific antigen (PSA) test is a blood test used to screen for prostate cancer in men. The test measures the levels of PSA, a protein produced by the prostate gland. Elevated PSA levels can indicate the presence of prostate cancer or other prostate conditions, such as benign prostatic hyperplasia (BPH) or prostatitis.

The PSA test is not a definitive test for prostate cancer and can produce false positive and false negative results. A positive PSA test result does not necessarily mean that a man has prostate cancer, and a negative result does not guarantee that a man is cancer-free. Therefore, further testing, such as a prostate biopsy, is typically required to confirm a diagnosis.

The use of PSA testing for prostate cancer screening remains controversial due to concerns over its accuracy and potential harm from unnecessary biopsies and treatments. The American Cancer Society recommends that men discuss the benefits and risks of PSA testing with their healthcare provider and make an informed decision about whether or not to be screened based on their individual risk factors and preferences.

In addition to the PSA test, other screening tests for prostate cancer include a digital rectal exam (DRE) and imaging tests such as an MRI or ultrasound. However, these tests are typically used in conjunction with PSA testing rather than as standalone screening methods.

Skin examination:

Skin examination is a type of cancer screening test that involves a visual inspection of the skin to check for any unusual or abnormal growths, moles, or lesions that may indicate skin cancer. This is particularly important for individuals who have a higher risk of developing skin cancer due to factors such as a family history of the disease, frequent sun exposure, fair skin, or a history of severe sunburns.

The skin examination typically involves a healthcare provider examining the skin over the entire body, including hard-to-see areas such as the scalp, back, and buttocks. The provider will look for any changes in the size, shape, color, or texture of moles or other skin growths, and may use a special magnifying lens or tool called a dermoscope to get a closer look at any suspicious areas.

If a suspicious lesion or growth is identified during the skin examination, a biopsy may be performed to determine whether it is cancerous. A biopsy involves removing a small sample of the tissue from the affected area and examining it under a microscope to look for cancer cells.

Regular skin examinations are important for early detection of skin cancer, as the earlier the cancer is detected, the better the chances for successful treatment and a positive outcome. Individuals should be aware of the signs and symptoms of skin cancer, such as changes in the appearance of moles or the development of new growths, and should report any concerns to their healthcare provider promptly. Additionally, individuals should protect their skin from sun damage by using sunscreen, wearing protective clothing, and avoiding prolonged exposure to the sun during peak hours.

Lung cancer screening:

Lung cancer screening is a process that involves using imaging tests to detect lung cancer at an early stage, before any symptoms become noticeable. The primary imaging test used for lung cancer screening is a low-dose computed tomography (LDCT) scan, which is a type of X-ray that uses low doses of radiation to create detailed images of the lungs.

The United States Preventive Services Task Force (USPSTF) recommends annual lung cancer screening for people who meet the following criteria:

- Are between the ages of 50 and 80

- Have a history of heavy smoking, defined as having smoked at least 30 pack-years (one pack per day for 30 years, two packs per day for 15 years, etc.)

- Are current smokers or have quit smoking within the past 15 years

The goal of lung cancer screening is to detect lung cancer at an early stage when it is more likely to be treatable. Studies have shown that lung cancer screening with LDCT can reduce the risk of dying from lung cancer by up to 20% in high-risk individuals.

It's important to note that not all lung nodules detected on a screening LDCT scan are cancerous. Many are benign, or non-cancerous, and do not require any treatment. However, if a nodule is suspicious for cancer, further testing such as a biopsy may be necessary to confirm the diagnosis.

If you are a current or former heavy smoker who meets the criteria for lung cancer screening, talk to your doctor about whether screening with LDCT is right for you.

It's important to note that the recommended screening guidelines may vary depending on an individual's age, gender, and personal or family medical history. It's best to consult with a healthcare professional to determine the appropriate screening schedule for you.

Chapter 7: Cancer Treatment and Survivorship

Chapter 7 of our guide focuses on cancer treatment and survivorship. Cancer treatment refers to the various methods used to manage or cure cancer, while survivorship is the period after treatment where cancer survivors are monitored for possible recurrence or side effects from their treatment. Advances in cancer treatment have led to improved outcomes and quality of life for cancer patients, and there are now a variety of treatment options available depending on the type and stage of cancer. This chapter will explore the different types of cancer treatment and the potential impact on survivorship, as well as strategies for managing post-treatment side effects and maintaining overall health and wellness.

Common cancer treatments

There are several types of cancer treatments available, and the most appropriate one(s) for a patient will depend on the type and stage of their cancer, as well as their overall health and preferences.

Some common cancer treatments include:

- Surgery: Surgery involves removing the cancerous tumor from the body. Depending on the type and stage of cancer, surgery may be the only treatment needed or may be combined with other treatments.

- Radiation therapy: Radiation therapy uses high-energy radiation to kill cancer cells. It can be delivered externally (from a machine outside the body) or internally (using radioactive materials placed inside the body).

- Chemotherapy: Chemotherapy uses drugs to kill cancer cells. These drugs can be given orally, through an IV, or injected directly into the cancerous area.

- Immunotherapy: Immunotherapy uses the body's own immune system to fight cancer. It can involve drugs that help the immune system identify and attack cancer cells, or treatments that use genetically modified immune cells.

- Hormone therapy: Hormone therapy is used to treat cancers that are sensitive to hormones, such as breast and prostate cancer. It involves blocking the hormones that fuel cancer growth.

- Targeted therapy: Targeted therapy uses drugs that specifically target the genetic mutations or other specific characteristics of cancer cells, while minimizing damage to healthy cells.

- Stem cell transplant: Stem cell transplant involves replacing damaged bone marrow (which produces blood cells) with healthy stem cells.

In addition to these treatments, clinical trials may also be an option for some patients. These trials test new treatments or combinations of treatments to determine their effectiveness and potential side effects.

Side effects of cancer treatment

While cancer treatments can be effective in targeting cancer cells and shrinking tumors, they can also cause side effects. The side effects of cancer treatment can vary depending on the type of treatment used, the dose and duration of treatment, and the individual's overall health.

Some common side effects of cancer treatment include fatigue, nausea, vomiting, diarrhea, hair loss, skin changes, mouth sores, and changes in appetite.
Chemotherapy and radiation therapy can also suppress the immune system, which can increase the risk of infections.

Other possible side effects of cancer treatment include neuropathy, or nerve damage, which can cause tingling, numbness, or pain in the hands and feet. Some cancer treatments can also cause fertility problems, sexual dysfunction, or hormonal imbalances. In some cases, cancer treatment can also cause long-term or late effects, such as increased risk of other cancers or chronic health conditions.

It's important for cancer patients to discuss potential side effects with their healthcare team before beginning treatment and to report any side effects that they experience during treatment. Healthcare providers can help manage side effects with medications, lifestyle changes, and other supportive therapies.

Strategies for coping with cancer treatment

Coping with cancer treatment can be challenging both physically and emotionally. The side effects of treatment such as fatigue, nausea, and hair loss can take a toll on the body, and the stress of coping with a cancer diagnosis and treatment can be overwhelming. However, there are several strategies that can help patients cope with these challenges:
- Seek support:

Practice self-care:

Physical, emotional, and mental well-being. Self-care can help you reduce stress, improve your quality of life, and cope better with the side effects of cancer treatment.

Some self-care strategies that can be helpful during cancer treatment include:

• Eating a healthy diet: Eating a balanced and nutritious diet can help you maintain your strength and energy, as well as support your immune system.

• Engaging in physical activity: Gentle exercise, such as walking or yoga, can help you maintain your strength and mobility, reduce stress, and improve your mood.

• Getting enough sleep: Getting enough rest is important for your physical and emotional health. Try to establish a regular sleep routine and create a relaxing sleep environment.

• Practicing relaxation techniques: Relaxation techniques, such as deep breathing, meditation, or guided imagery, can help reduce stress, anxiety, and pain.

• Seeking social support: Talking to friends, family, or a support group can help you feel less isolated and provide you with emotional support.

• Managing your emotions: It is normal to experience a range of emotions during cancer treatment, including fear, anxiety, and sadness. Finding healthy ways to express and cope with these emotions, such as through journaling or talking to a counselor, can help you manage your emotional well-being.

• Taking breaks: It is important to take breaks from cancer treatment and make time for activities you enjoy, such as reading a book, watching a movie, or spending time with loved ones. These activities can help you relax and take your mind off cancer treatment.

Utilize stress-reducing techniques:

Cancer treatment can be physically and emotionally challenging, and patients may experience a range of stress-related symptoms such as anxiety, depression, and fatigue. To cope with these challenges, patients are encouraged to utilize stress-reducing techniques that can help improve their quality of life.

One of the most effective stress-reducing techniques for cancer patients is mindfulness meditation. This practice involves focusing your attention on the present moment without judgment, allowing you to cultivate a sense of calm and awareness. Research has shown that mindfulness meditation can help reduce symptoms of anxiety, depression, and fatigue in cancer patients.

Other stress-reducing techniques include deep breathing exercises, progressive muscle relaxation, and guided imagery. These techniques can help promote relaxation and reduce stress by calming the mind and body. Additionally, engaging in regular physical activity, such as gentle yoga or walking, can also help reduce stress and improve overall well-being.

It's important to work with your healthcare team to develop an individualized plan for managing stress during cancer treatment. This may include counseling or other forms of therapy, as well as medication to manage symptoms like anxiety or depression. By incorporating stress-reducing techniques into your daily routine, you can help alleviate some of the emotional burdens associated with cancer treatment and improve your overall quality of life.

Engage in hobbies and activities:

Engaging in hobbies and activities can be a helpful strategy for coping with cancer treatment. Cancer treatment can be emotionally and physically draining, so participating in enjoyable activities can provide a much-needed break and a sense of normalcy. Hobbies and activities can also provide a sense of accomplishment and boost self-esteem, which can be helpful during a challenging time.

Examples of hobbies and activities that cancer patients may find enjoyable include reading, gardening, painting, playing music, knitting, writing, or participating in a sport or exercise program. It's important to find activities that are enjoyable and achievable, and to not put too much pressure on oneself to be perfect or productive. The goal of engaging in hobbies and activities during cancer treatment is to provide a distraction from the stress of treatment and to provide a sense of enjoyment and fulfillment.

Participating in social activities and spending time with loved ones can be especially helpful for cancer patients. Connecting with others who understand what you're going through can provide a sense of community and support. It can also be helpful to seek out support groups or online forums for cancer patients to connect with others who are going through similar experiences.

Communicate with healthcare providers:

Effective communication with healthcare providers is essential for successful cancer treatment and survivorship. Open and honest communication can help ensure that patients receive the best possible care and support throughout their cancer journey.

Here are some ways to effectively communicate with healthcare providers:

- Be honest about your symptoms and concerns: It is essential to be honest with your healthcare provider about any symptoms or concerns you may have. This can help them provide appropriate treatment and support.

- Ask questions: Don't hesitate to ask questions if you are unclear about any aspect of your cancer treatment or care. Ask your healthcare provider to explain any medical terms or procedures you may not understand.

- Keep a record: It can be helpful to keep a record of your symptoms, treatments, and medications. This information can help you keep track of your progress and communicate effectively with your healthcare provider.

- Bring a support person: Consider bringing a trusted family member or friend to appointments. They can help you remember important details and ask questions on your behalf.

- Be proactive: Take an active role in your cancer care by educating yourself about your diagnosis and treatment options. This can help you make informed decisions and communicate more effectively with your healthcare provider.

By practicing effective communication with healthcare providers, cancer patients can feel more in control of their treatment and improve their chances of successful treatment and survivorship.

Consider complementary therapies:

Complementary therapies are therapies that are used in addition to conventional medical treatments. They are also sometimes called integrative therapies. Some complementary therapies may help people manage the side effects of cancer treatment, while others may be used to improve overall well-being.

Examples of complementary therapies include acupuncture, massage therapy, meditation, yoga, and nutritional supplements. These therapies can help reduce stress and anxiety, improve mood, and relieve pain and nausea. They can also help improve sleep quality and energy levels, which can be particularly important during cancer treatment.

It is important to note that not all complementary therapies are safe or effective, and some may interact with cancer treatments or other medications. It is important to speak with your healthcare provider before starting any complementary therapy. They can help you understand the potential benefits and risks, and can work with you to develop a safe and effective plan that complements your cancer treatment plan.

Ccoping with cancer treatment involves a combination of physical self-care, emotional support, and effective communication with healthcare providers.

Life after cancer treatment

After completing cancer treatment, many people find that they face a new set of challenges as they adjust to life after treatment. While this can be a time of celebration and relief, it can also be a period of uncertainty and fear.

One of the primary concerns for cancer survivors is the fear of recurrence. This fear can be especially strong in the months following treatment, as survivors adjust to life without the constant medical attention and monitoring that was a part of their treatment process. It is important for survivors to talk to their healthcare providers about their fears and to develop a follow-up care plan that includes regular monitoring and check-ups.

Survivors may also struggle with physical and emotional changes related to their cancer and its treatment. These changes can include fatigue, pain, loss of appetite, weight gain or loss, and changes in sexual function. Survivors may also experience anxiety, depression, or other mental health concerns. It is important for survivors to be open and honest with their healthcare providers about these changes and to seek support from friends, family members, and mental health professionals as needed.

In addition to addressing physical and emotional changes, survivors may also face practical challenges related to their employment, finances, and relationships. Some survivors may need to make changes to their work schedule or take time off to deal with ongoing treatment or recovery. Financial challenges may also arise, as medical bills and other expenses related to cancer treatment can be significant. Survivors may benefit from seeking support from financial counselors, social workers, or other professionals who can help them navigate these challenges.

Many survivors find that they benefit from connecting with other survivors and participating in support groups or other survivorship programs. These resources can provide emotional support, practical guidance, and a sense of community to help survivors adjust to life after cancer treatment.

Cancer survivorship and follow-up care

Cancer survivorship refers to the period of time after cancer treatment has ended and the person is in remission or has no evidence of disease. While this can be a time of celebration and relief, it can also be a time of adjustment and uncertainty. Follow-up care is an important part of survivorship, as it helps to monitor for any signs of cancer recurrence, manage long-term side effects of treatment, and provide support for the emotional and psychological impact of cancer.

The specific follow-up care recommended for each individual will depend on the type of cancer they had, the stage of the cancer, and the type of treatment received. However, some general guidelines include regular check-ups with a primary care physician or oncologist, routine imaging or blood tests, and screening for other health issues that may arise due to cancer treatment (such as heart disease or osteoporosis).

In addition to medical follow-up, cancer survivors may also benefit from other types of support. This can include counseling or therapy to address the emotional and psychological impact of cancer, support groups to connect with others who have had similar experiences, and lifestyle changes to promote overall health and well-being.

It is important for cancer survivors to continue to prioritize their health and well-being after treatment ends. This may include adopting healthy lifestyle habits such as regular exercise, a balanced diet, and avoiding tobacco and excessive alcohol consumption. It is also important to communicate with healthcare providers about any concerns or symptoms that arise, as early detection and treatment of any issues can help to promote long-term health and well-being.

Chapter 8: Additional Strategies for Cancer Prevention

Chapter 8 focuses on additional strategies for cancer prevention, beyond the lifestyle changes and screening discussed in previous chapters. While there is no guaranteed way to prevent cancer, there are steps that can be taken to reduce the risk of developing the disease. This chapter explores various approaches to cancer prevention, including vaccinations, chemoprevention, and genetic testing. Additionally, the chapter emphasizes the importance of staying informed about cancer prevention research and seeking professional medical advice when making decisions about personal health.

Immunizations for cancer prevention

Immunizations are an important strategy for cancer prevention. Certain vaccines can help prevent viral infections that are known to increase the risk of certain types of cancer. For example, the human papillomavirus (HPV) vaccine can help prevent HPV infection, which is a major cause of cervical cancer, as well as several other types of cancer, such as anal cancer, penile cancer, and oropharyngeal cancer. The hepatitis B vaccine can also help prevent hepatitis B infection, which can lead to liver cancer.

It's important to note that these vaccines are most effective when administered before the onset of sexual activity or exposure to hepatitis B, respectively. Therefore, the HPV vaccine is typically recommended for boys and girls between the ages of 11 and 12, while the hepatitis B vaccine is recommended for infants, children, and adolescents, as well as certain high-risk adults.

Other vaccines, such as the influenza vaccine and pneumococcal vaccine, can also help prevent infections that can weaken the immune system and increase the risk of cancer. For example, people with weakened immune systems due to cancer treatment may be at increased risk of developing infections such as pneumonia, which can be prevented by the pneumococcal vaccine. It's important to talk to your healthcare provider about which vaccines may be appropriate for you based on your individual risk factors and medical history.

Quitting smoking and other tobacco products

Quitting smoking and other tobacco products is one of the most important steps a person can take to prevent cancer. Tobacco smoke contains more than 70 known carcinogens, which are substances that are capable of causing cancer. These carcinogens can damage the DNA in cells and lead to the development of cancer.

Smoking is a major risk factor for several types of cancer, including lung, throat, mouth, bladder, kidney, pancreas, and cervical cancer. Secondhand smoke can also increase the risk of lung cancer in non-smokers.

Quitting smoking and other tobacco products can greatly reduce a person's risk of developing cancer. In fact, the risk of lung cancer decreases by about 50% within 10 years of quitting smoking. Other benefits of quitting include improved lung function, reduced risk of heart disease and stroke, and better overall health.

There are many different methods for quitting smoking, including nicotine replacement therapy, prescription medications, and behavioral counseling. It's important for individuals to find a method that works best for them and to seek support from healthcare providers, family, and friends.

It's also important to note that quitting smoking is not only beneficial for preventing cancer, but it can also have a positive impact on the health of those around the individual who quits. Secondhand smoke can cause cancer and other health problems in non-smokers, so quitting smoking can help protect others from the harmful effects of tobacco smoke.

Limiting alcohol consumption

Limiting alcohol consumption is an important strategy for cancer prevention. According to the American Cancer Society, there is a strong link between alcohol consumption and an increased risk of developing several types of cancer, including breast, liver, colon, and esophageal cancer. Alcohol consumption is believed to damage DNA, increase estrogen levels in women, and lead to liver damage, all of which can increase the risk of cancer.

To reduce the risk of cancer, the American Cancer Society recommends limiting alcohol consumption to no more than one drink per day for women and no more than two drinks per day for men. It's also important to note that binge drinking, which is defined as consuming four or more drinks in one sitting for women and five or more drinks for men, can increase the risk of cancer even more.

If you are struggling to limit your alcohol consumption, there are several strategies that may be helpful. These include setting limits on the amount of alcohol you consume, avoiding situations where you are likely to drink excessively, and seeking support from friends, family members, or a healthcare professional. Additionally, it's important to be aware of the signs of alcohol addiction and seek treatment if necessary.

Sleep hygiene and cancer prevention

Sleep hygiene refers to a set of habits and practices that promote good sleep quality and quantity. Getting sufficient high-quality sleep is essential for overall health and well-being, and research has shown that poor sleep habits may increase the risk of certain types of cancer.

Studies have shown that individuals who regularly experience poor sleep quality or insufficient sleep have a higher risk of developing breast, prostate, and colorectal cancer. This is thought to be due to disruptions in the body's circadian rhythms, which can affect the production of hormones and other physiological processes that play a role in cancer development.

To promote good sleep hygiene and reduce the risk of cancer, it is recommended to establish a regular sleep schedule and stick to it as closely as possible, avoid caffeine and alcohol close to bedtime, create a relaxing sleep environment that is free of distractions, and limit exposure to screens and other stimulating activities before bed.

In addition to these habits, it is also important to address any underlying sleep disorders, such as sleep apnea or insomnia, through medical treatment or behavioral therapy. By taking steps to improve sleep hygiene, individuals can support their overall health and reduce their risk of cancer.

Conclusion

As we reach the end of this guide, it is important to reflect on the information presented about cancer prevention and management. Cancer is a complex disease with many different risk factors and potential treatments. However, by adopting healthy lifestyle habits, utilizing screening tests, and following medical advice, individuals can take proactive steps to reduce their risk of developing cancer or improve their chances of successful treatment and survivorship. In this conclusion, we will summarize some key takeaways from this guide and emphasize the importance of continued efforts to prevent and manage cancer.

Summarize the key points:

here's a summary of the key points covered in this guide:

Chapter 1: Understanding Cancer
- Cancer is a complex disease caused by abnormal cell growth and division.
- There are many different types of cancer, each with its own characteristics and risk factors.
- Early detection and prompt treatment can improve outcomes and increase the chances of a successful recovery.

Chapter 2: Cancer Risk Factors
- Certain lifestyle factors, such as tobacco use, alcohol consumption, poor diet, and lack of physical activity, can increase the risk of developing cancer.
- Other factors, such as genetics, age, and environmental exposures, can also contribute to cancer risk.
- Understanding and addressing these risk factors can help reduce the chances of developing cancer.

Chapter 3: Nutrition and Cancer Prevention
- Eating a balanced diet that includes a variety of fruits, vegetables, whole grains, and lean proteins can help reduce the risk of cancer.
- Certain foods and nutrients, such as cruciferous vegetables, berries, and omega-3 fatty acids, may have particular cancer-fighting properties.
- Avoiding processed foods, red meat, and excessive amounts of alcohol can also help lower cancer risk.

Chapter 4: Physical Activity and Cancer Prevention
- Regular exercise can help reduce the risk of several types of cancer, as well as improve overall health and wellbeing.
- Aim for at least 150 minutes of moderate-intensity activity or 75 minutes of vigorous-intensity activity per week.
- Incorporating strength training and flexibility exercises can also be beneficial.

Chapter 5: Stress Management
- Chronic stress can weaken the immune system and contribute to the development of cancer.
- Mindfulness practices, such as meditation and yoga, can help reduce stress and promote relaxation.
- Other stress-reducing techniques include exercise, social support, time management, and cognitive-behavioral therapy.

Chapter 6: Cancer Screening and Early Detection
- Regular cancer screenings can help detect cancer early, when it is most treatable.
- Guidelines for cancer screening vary depending on age, sex, and individual risk factors.
- Screening tests may include mammography, colonoscopy, Pap test, PSA test, skin examination, and lung cancer screening.

Chapter 7: Cancer Treatment and Survivorship
- Common cancer treatments include surgery, chemotherapy, radiation therapy, immunotherapy, and targeted therapy.
- These treatments can cause a variety of side effects, which can be managed with self-care, stress-reducing techniques, and complementary therapies.
- After treatment, survivors may face ongoing physical and emotional challenges, and should receive regular follow-up care to monitor for potential cancer recurrence.

Chapter 8: Additional Strategies for Cancer Prevention
- Immunizations, such as the HPV vaccine, can help prevent certain types of cancer.
- Avoiding tobacco use and limiting alcohol consumption can also lower cancer risk.
- Maintaining good sleep hygiene and reducing exposure to environmental toxins may also be beneficial.

Emphasize the importance of cancer prevention:

Cancer prevention is a critical aspect of overall health and wellbeing. It is essential to note that many cancers can be prevented by making healthy lifestyle choices and reducing exposure to risk factors. Prevention strategies include avoiding tobacco and limiting alcohol consumption, maintaining a healthy weight, engaging in regular physical activity, protecting the skin from excessive sun exposure, getting vaccinated against cancer-causing viruses, and participating in cancer screening programs for early detection. By implementing these strategies, individuals can significantly reduce their risk of developing cancer and improve their chances of leading a long and healthy life.

Encourage action:

Encouraging action is a crucial component of any discussion about cancer prevention and management. It is not enough to simply acknowledge the importance of prevention measures and early detection; individuals must take action to protect their health. Encouraging action can involve providing specific recommendations for lifestyle changes or screening tests, as well as offering resources and support for individuals to make those changes. It can also involve addressing barriers to action, such as fear or lack of access to healthcare. Encouraging action can be accomplished through targeted education campaigns, community outreach programs, and individual counseling and support. Ultimately, it is through action that we can make progress in the fight against cancer.

Cancer is a disease that affects millions of people worldwide and has a significant impact on both patients and their families. While there is no guaranteed way to prevent cancer, there are many strategies that individuals can adopt to reduce their risk and improve their overall health. In this book, we have explored a variety of approaches to cancer prevention, screening, and treatment.

One of the key takeaways from this book is the importance of lifestyle factors in cancer prevention. Adopting healthy habits such as regular exercise, a balanced diet, and avoiding tobacco and excessive alcohol consumption can significantly reduce an individual's risk of developing cancer. Additionally, cancer screening can detect cancer at an early stage when it is most treatable, increasing the likelihood of successful treatment and survival.

In discussing cancer treatment, we highlighted the various treatment options available to patients, including surgery, radiation therapy, chemotherapy, and targeted therapy. While these treatments can be effective in fighting cancer, they can also have significant side effects. We also explored coping strategies for patients undergoing cancer treatment, including self-care, stress reduction techniques, and complementary therapies.

We emphasized the importance of follow-up care and survivorship after cancer treatment. Regular check-ups and monitoring can detect any potential recurrence or side effects of treatment, and survivors can benefit from support groups and resources designed to address the unique challenges they face.

It is clear that cancer prevention and treatment are complex topics that require a multifaceted approach. It is important for individuals to take responsibility for their health and adopt healthy habits to reduce their risk of developing cancer. Equally important is access to high-quality cancer screening and treatment for those who do develop the disease. With continued research and education, we can make progress in the fight against cancer.

The information presented in this book underscores the importance of cancer prevention, screening, and treatment. By taking action to reduce our risk of cancer, staying vigilant with regular screenings, and utilizing the most effective treatment options available, we can work towards a future where cancer is no longer a devastating disease. It is my hope that this book has provided valuable insights and resources for those affected by cancer, as well as their loved ones, caregivers, and healthcare providers.